Animals as the Third in Relational Psychotherapy

Animals as the Third in Relational Psychotherapy: Exploring Theory, Frame and Practice elegantly and skilfully weaves together relevant literature, clinical reflections, compelling case material and contemporary psychoanalytic theory to demonstrate how the presence of an animal in the treatment arena can eventually bring about relational, interpersonal and intrapsychic change.

Contemporary relational psychoanalytic literature has been virtually silent about our relationship with animals, a feature seemingly intrinsic to our relational worlds. This book seeks to remediate this void by giving voice to the practice and principles of working relationally in the presence of an animal. The text accentuates recurrent themes: animals are seen by human beings as significant subjective others and are treated as legitimate partners for relational and interpersonal processes, attachment figures and transferential objects; animals in the psychotherapy environment can play the role as a 'bridge' from the unconscious to the conscious, from the dissociated to the experienced, from the intrapsychic to the interpersonal; as the third in the treatment arena, the animal helps to reveal the field, bringing conflicts to life and making them available for analysis in the clinical setting.

In seeking to authorise the incorporation of animals into the practice of relational psychotherapy the text applies conventional concepts to novel contexts; it extends psychoanalytic and relational principles to create a theoretical framework within which to consider the therapeutic effects of working in the triadic interactions of therapist, client and animal and thus also begins to evolve a new version of relational psychoanalytic practice. The authors value the human-animal experience in treatment and repeatedly show how the application of a relational psychoanalytic lens to the patient-therapist-animal triad can enhance the therapeutic process in ways that encourage progressive communication, understanding of the patient and the relaxing of defences, leading to the symbolising of relational capacity, therapeutic breakthrough and intrapsychic change.

Jo Silbert has worked in South Africa, Zimbabwe and Australia as a social worker, counsellor, psychotherapist and trainer in the educational, public, private and NGO sectors. She is interested in interpersonal neurobiology, mindfulness and in issues of social justice. Jo is currently involved in editing and writing.

Jo Frasca is a psychotherapist in private practice in Sydney, Australia, working with adults, adolescents and couples. She works within the psychoanalytic relational frame and is interested in public education on the differing professional services offered for emotional and mental health. This is Jo's second book and she is currently working on a third.

Animals as the Third in Relational Psychotherapy

Exploring Theory, Frame and Practice

Edited by Jo Silbert and Jo Frasca

Routledge
Taylor & Francis Group

LONDON AND NEW YORK

First published 2021
by Routledge
2 Park Square, Milton Park, Abingdon, Oxon OX14 4RN

and by Routledge
52 Vanderbilt Avenue, New York, NY 10017

Routledge is an imprint of the Taylor & Francis Group, an informa business

British Library Cataloguing-in-Publication Data
A catalogue record for this book is available from the British Library

Library of Congress Cataloging-in-Publication Data
A catalog record has been requested for this book

ISBN: 978-0-367-43778-7 (hbk)
ISBN: 978-0-367-43780-0 (pbk)
ISBN: 978-1-003-00573-5 (ebk)

Typeset in Times New Roman
by codeMantra

Contents

Acknowledgements

To our families, friends and colleagues, for their sustenance, help, scrutiny and wisdom and whose clarity, rigour and knowledge challenged us and brought coherence, depth and complexity to our work;

to our contributors, for their tenacity in hanging in with us through a complex and sometimes challenging process over an extended period and whose questions, contributions and passion helped to make this book all the more bountiful;

to our patients, for their courage and perseverance and whose responses to the animals in their therapy spaces and treatment processes encouraged us to embrace new possibilities, extended us and opened our hearts and minds to the breadth, richness and uniqueness of their internal and relational worlds;

to our non-human companions, for accompanying us into unfamiliar territory and who, by their loyalty and lack of judgement, tested us, taught us and supported our work by their presence and with qualities which we are privileged to have experienced and have yet fully to understand;

to you all, we extend our sincere and heartfelt thanks

Contributor biographies

Joanne Emmens is a psychoanalytic psychotherapist and lecturer teaching at AUT University in Auckland, New Zealand, and in private practice. She teaches psychoanalytic theory and practice to psychotherapy master's students and supervises academic dissertations. Joanne specialises in working with complex trauma, psychotic disturbance and dissociative disorders.

Affiliations:
New Zealand Association of Psychotherapists (NZAP)
Psychotherapy Board of Aotearoa NewZealand (PBANZ)

Beth Feldman is a clinical psychologist in private practice for over twenty-five years, has a PhD in clinical psychology from Long Island University and became a Certified Psychoanalyst after training at The Suffolk Institute for Psychotherapy and Psychoanalysis. She has advanced training in the treatment of Addictions and Eating Disorders and is the proud parent of three canines and two humans.

Affiliations:
American Psychological Association
The Nassau County Psychological Association
The Suffolk Institute of Psychotherapy and Psychoanalysis.

Gaiana Germani, PhD, is a practicing psychoanalyst. After completing her doctorate in Clinical Psychology at the University of Massachusetts in 2002, she lectured at Harvard Medical School, served as President of the Massachusetts Association for Psychoanalytic Psychotherapy, and completed her psychoanalytic training in 2020 at the Massachusetts Institute for Psychoanalysis.

Affiliations:
Massachusetts Institute for Psychoanalysis
Society for Psychoanalysis and Psychoanalytic Psychology – Division 39 – American Psychological Association

Gretchen Heyer, PhD, is a training analyst with the Interregional Society of Jungian Analysts. Her essays and articles have appeared in psychology and literary journals. She grew up in remote areas of Africa and maintains a private practice in Houston.

Affiliations:
> International Association of Relational Psychoanalysts and Psychotherapists
> Society for Psychoanalysis and Psychoanalytic Psychology Division 39
> International Association of Analytical Psychology
> Interregional Society of Jungian Analysts
> Houston Psychoanalytic Society

Lynn Higgins, LCSW, has been working as a psychoanalyst with children, adolescents and adults in private practice. She is interested in the connection between mind/body and the neuropsychology of the psyche.

Affiliations:
> New York State Society of Clinical Social Workers, Nassau/Suffolk Chapter
> International Association of Relational Psychoanalytic Psychotherapy
> American Psychological Association: Division 39
> American Association of Psychoanalytic Clinical Social Workers
> National Association of Social Workers, New York City Chapter
> New York State Psychological Association
> Suffolk Institute for Psychoanalysis and Psychotherapy
> American Dance Therapy Association

Sean Meggeson holds a diploma in Relational Psychotherapy from *The Toronto Institute for Relational Psychotherapy* and is a graduate of The William Alanson White Institute Intensive Psychoanalytic Psychotherapy Program. He has lectured on a variety of topics including Jacques Lacan and James Joyce, working intimately with addiction, and alternative rock music.

Affiliations:
> Registered Psychotherapist with the College of Registered Psychotherapists of Ontario
> Guest member of the *Toronto Psychoanalytic Society.*
> Member of *The International Association for Relational Psychoanalysis and Psychotherapy*

Virginia Rachmani is a psychotherapist and psychoanalyst having graduated from New York University. She is in private practice in Manhattan, serves as a supervisor and faculty member at the National Institute for the Psychotherapies and the American Institute of Psychoanalysis and on the board of the *American Journal of Psychoanalysis.*

Affiliations:
> National Institute for the Psychotherapies
> American Institute of Psychoanalysis

Dor Roitman was born and raised in Israel, and lived most of his childhood on a Kibbutz, before serving in the IAF as a co-pilot. He trained simultaneously as an animal-assisted therapist and as a clinical psychologist and later completed training as a group analyst. He works in a private clinic and in the Jaffa Community Centre for Mental Health Services.

Affiliations:
Israeli Association of Animal-Assisted Psychotherapy (IAAAP)
Israeli Institute of Group Analysis (IIGP).
Jaffa Community Center for Mental Health Services (NHS.

David Vincent is a Group Analyst, a Psychoanalytic Psychotherapist and an Interpersonal Therapist and Supervisor (IPT). He has a Doctorate from the Centre for Psychoanalytic Studies at Essex University. He was a Consultant Adult Psychotherapist at Forest House Clinic (NHS) and is now retired.

Affiliations:
A retired member of the Institute of Group Analysis (London) and the British Psychotherapy Foundation

1   Rat Man to relationality

An introduction

Jo Silbert

The jealous and violent Titan Kronos, son of Zeus, was enraged. He was unaccustomed to being ignored. Yet his advances had been rejected by the beautiful sea nymph, Philyra. Seething and scheming, he plotted his revenge. With his supernatural powers he turned himself into a stallion, relentlessly pursued the unsuspecting Philyra, and brutally raped her.

From this savage and violent union, Chiron was conceived.

Being the child of a supreme deity, Chiron, was born immortal. And in a cruel embodiment of his traumatic conception, he was also born a centaur, a creature with the torso of a human male and the hind legs of a horse. Philyra was repulsed by Chiron, perhaps due to his deformity, perhaps in anticipation of the onset of depraved behaviour for which centaurs were notorious, perhaps for reflecting an aspect of her own history that was unbearable for her. As nine months earlier she had rejected his father, Philyra abandoned her baby.

Before long, the supreme god, Apollo, god of defence and destruction, of poetry and music, of archery and healing, rescued and adopted the infant. At Apollo's feet, Chiron was exposed to the arts, sciences, medicine and morality and although a centaur in form, grew up to be utterly unlike his centaur counterparts in substance.

Centaurs were known to be lascivious, hedonistic, rowdy and deviant, but not Chiron. Chiron developed into a wise and esteemed teacher of morality, an astrologer, a gifted healer, a mentor, a bridge between the world of humans and that of animals, much-loved and widely respected.

Amongst Chiron's cohort of illustrious students was the god Hercules. One evening over dinner and a bottle of sacred wine, Hercules and Chiron suddenly found themselves surrounded by a mob of marauding, menacing centaurs who had been attracted by the smell of the alcohol. The centaurs attacked. Hercules in defence of Chiron and himself, counter-attacked with his arrows, killing many of the centaurs.

Perhaps it was a stray arrow, perhaps Hercules mistook the centaur Chiron for one of their assailants, but one of Hercules' arrows, made all the more lethal by a serpent's venom and meant for their aggressors, accidentally struck his gentle and beloved teacher and friend.

Chiron was critically injured and in agony. He mustered up his superior healing powers but was rendered impotent. It was not possible for the wounded healer to heal himself and, despite yearning for death to release him from his distress, it was also not possible for a deity to die. With his wounds unattended, he was destined to endure excruciating torment in perpetuity.

Meanwhile, Prometheus, supreme trickster and god of fire, having angered the gods by stealing fire from them, had been banished to Mount Olympus where he was being punished in eternal horror by having his liver devoured by an eagle. As a deity, Prometheus too was destined to live forever, and like Chiron continued to suffer in tortured despair, from a cruel alliance of injury and immortality.

Vanquished by relentless pain, desperate to be liberated by death, Chiron devised a plan. If Hercules would agree to exchange his own mortality for Chiron's immortality, Chiron would offer to change places with Prometheus, thereby freeing Prometheus from his torture, bestowing perpetual life upon him and conferring upon Hercules an opportunity for him to simultaneously liberate his unintended victim, redeem himself and live forever.

And so it transpired. Hercules gave his mortality to Chiron in exchange for eternal life, Chiron took Prometheus's place on Mount Olympus and Prometheus was liberated from his excruciating fate. With his own liver being devoured by the eagle, the now-mortal Chiron waited to surrender to death.

As Apollo had rescued the infant Chiron, his grandfather Zeus now took pity on him, and freed Chiron, half-man half-animal, gifted and wounded healer, supreme being, into the heavens to be immortalised, after all, as a star.

Animals have always occupied a significant place in the lives of humans, initially as food, as a means of transport, and as companions for some 15,000 years (Beck, 2000). Our relationship with animals, however, is richer and more complex than one based only on their utilitarian value or on the comfort they offer to humans. Animals have forever been grafted into the human psyche. They appear in cave drawings and art throughout the ages, in stellar constellations, like zodiac signs, and in mythology and fairy tales, and are integral to polytheism, shamanism, traditional faiths, and contemporary religious life (von Buchholtz, 2000).

Animals in psychoanalysis

According to Freud, animals, in some form, have crawled, crept, leapt, trotted, hopped, slithered, swum, flown, or flittered their way into psychoanalytic literature.

In Freud's later writings, we learn of his well-known love of and devotion to his dogs that entered his life and his therapy room in his later years. We discover his belief about their perceptiveness regarding the emotional landscape of his patients, the calming and comforting effect they had on both him and those he was treating, and their intuition about the end of sessions.

But much earlier on in his work, we are introduced to a unique portrayal of human-animal relationships (Suen, 2013). In *Totem and Taboo*, Freud (2001) argues that, given their parents' tendency to manage human sexuality by obscuring, denying, fictionalising, or romanticising the facts, children perceive themselves as less like their parents and far more akin to animals, in their shared lack of both arrogance and inhibition about their bodily functions. Animals, he suggests, were thus far more useful to children as objects of childhood observation in the development of their theories of sexuality. He observes that at some point, however, a child will suddenly develop a phobia about an animal to which she or he was hitherto attached – 'a very common, and perhaps the earliest, form of psychoneurotic illness' (p. 147). It is thus that animals play a role in the gathering of material for the formation of the oedipus complex. And it is thus that animals come to enter the dreams of his child patients.

Freud's exploration and analysis of the dreams of his child patients offers his most detailed consideration of animal-human relationships (De Chavez, 2015). His focus on infantile neuroses in *The Rat Man: Notes upon a case of obsessional neurosis* and *The Wolf Man: From a history of an infantile neurosis* reveals the intrapsychic centrality of the imaginal animal (ibid) as representative of oedipal desire. Other than in his consideration of the androgynous vulture in Leonardo da Vinci's dream which, as mother-substitute, has an empowering effect on da Vinci as a child (ibid), Freud proposes that, in his child patients' dreams, the punitive father, manifesting as the feared animal, threatens castration as punishment for the child's sexual desire for the mother and death-wish for the father. The animal for Freud is thus seen as an intrapsychic representative of drives, and the task of analysis is to interrogate the dream material in order to excavate its latent content.

Freud further extends the reference to animals in *Totem and Taboo*. While it is beyond the scope of this chapter to elaborate upon these ideas, it is worth noting that in his endeavour to determine an anthropological predisposition for the oedipus complex, he attempts to establish a link between the infantile anxiety triggered by animals and the ambivalent status of the 'totem' animal in the so-called primitive societies (Marinelli and Mayer, 2016).

Much later on in Freud's work, his interest in animals turned to observations of domestic animals in both his life and his treatment room; when he was in his 70s, he met Wolf, 'an Alsatian shepherd with a wide grin and bat-like ears and just like that, dogs went from being Freudian symbols to being Freudian friends and office mates' (Freud in Braitman, 2014).

Reflecting with great affection and tenderness on the influence upon his patients of his first Chow, Jofi, he wrote, 'a charming creature, so interesting in her feminine characteristics too, wild, impulsive, intelligent' (ibid). He noticed that both he and his patients were calmer in Jofi's presence (Coren, 2013), which, he suggested, softened resistance and enabled his patients to more easily disclose difficult material, thereby facilitating the analysis. He wrote movingly of the enormous comfort his dogs were to him personally, at times of distress, illness, loss, and impending death.

Molnar (1996) points out an interesting tension in Freud's considerations of the animal presence. The theoretical discourse of the oedipus complex contends that in dream content, the feared animal, as a substitute for the punitive father, is a sign of neurotic ambivalence; his companion dogs, on the other hand, are imbued with positive qualities, which he experiences as objects of attachment, as feminine, and as encouraging the therapeutic process. In exploring this idea, Suen (2013) proposes that perhaps we are

> willing to speak, and speak even the most difficult truth, when we see the animal not as a fearful, punitive creature, but rather as a maternal figure to whom we look for support and inspiration when we have momentarily lost our voice (p. 137).

Several further ironies are embedded in Freud's hypotheses about human-animal relationships. Neither Freud nor his followers tried to analyse animals or their relationships with humans (see Brown's 2004 paper, *The Human-Animal Bond and Self Psychology: Toward a New Understanding* as an example of the utilising psychoanalytic theory for such an exploration) nor, once animals had been introduced into Freud's consulting room, did he consider their representational role in the analytic process. Given that the oedipus complex is a theory anchored in the familial, social, and religious structures of a patriarchal society (Suen, 2013), Roitman (2018, personal communication) attributes this omission, in part, to the experience of the human-animal bond being predicated upon the then-dominant Western belief in the superiority of humans over 'wild and bestial' animals. At the time, Freud noted in *Totem and Taboo* that animals were perceived to be more akin to children and members of pre-literate societies, and similarly needed to be subjugated and tamed. Indeed, Myers (in Serpell, 1999) and Deleuze and Guattari (in De Chavez, 2015) criticise Freudian theory for its tendency to reduce animals to symbols or disguised impulses. Nevertheless, this clarification may also help to justify why, despite Freud's work on transference, it was his daughter Anna, rather than Freud himself, who speculated about the transferential relationship between her father and his canine companions, when she jokingly suggested that he transferred his affection for her onto his dogs (Braitman, 2014).

As conspicuous, albeit defensible, as these omissions are, the matter did not end there. In the early 1960s, Freud's writing about his companion dogs subsequently became the basis for the launching of a system of animal-assisted therapeutic interventions that deviated from a psychoanalytical orientation and veered towards prioritising the remedial potential of the human-animal bond in health promotion and cognitive and behavioural change (Bachi and Parish-Plass, 2016; Brown, 2004; Kruger and Serpell, 2010). Some of the features of animal-assisted therapy will be elaborated upon later in this chapter. Prior to this elaboration, a brief reference to animals in the work of Ferenczi, Rank, Hermann, and Jung is merited.

Following Freud, Ferenczi and Rank continued to reference animals in their work, although later digressed in their focus from their predecessor's interpretation of the symbolism of animals in the oedipal complex. Rank extended the scope of the oedipal complex, asserting that infantile animal phobias were also linked to the trauma of birth and represented the child's unconscious wish to return to the mother's womb. Ferenczi, motivating for a return to hypnosis as the preferred psychoanalytic technique, argued that the imagined animal revealed the child's attachment to both parents (Marinelli and Mayer, 2016).

Although animals continued to feature marginally in psychoanalytic literature as in the work of the authors mentioned above, Marinelli and Mayer (ibid.) assert that most of the work involving animals did not, in the main, enhance the formulation of psychoanalytic theory nor deepen our understanding of the scope of the human-animal bond for therapeutic outcome. They draw our attention, however, to the work of the more peripheral Imre Hermann, whose contribution, they argue, does meaningfully progress psychoanalytic thinking.

Initially trained as an experimental psychologist, Hermann's training analysis awakened in him an interest in a comparative study of human and animal behaviour. His investigation of primatology and animal psychology, despite his methodology being criticised for its reliance on indirect observation, contributed notably to a major shift in psychoanalytic theory from the classical triangular oedipal model towards attachment theories, which instead highlighted the pre-oedipal stage and the mother-child dyad. Marinelli and Mayer (ibid) contend that Hermann's work is thus salient in its demonstration of the transition from, and reformulation of, Freud's hypotheses about the nature of instincts to a more ethologically informed approach in which animals feature. The psychoanalytic reception of animal psychology in the 1920s, albeit by indirect observation, thus predated the actual observation of children and babies, as practiced by Klein and later attachment theorists such as Spitz or Bowlby (ibid) and perhaps even pioneered observation as a viable method for the gathering of data for analysis.

Jung's work on the role of animals also adds materially to the literature. Underpinned by his religious conviction, his love and admiration of animals, and his 'unconscious identity' (Jung, 1995, p. 121) with them, he deviated from both the dominant ideological discourse which, at the time of his writing, attributed a lower status to animals than humans, and from the dominant trends in psychoanalytic theory. While he and Freud and his followers believed that the imagined animal provides useful information about a patient's unconscious material, Jung's beliefs that animals are superior to humans (Hannah, 2006) and are representative of the 'divine' dimension of the human psyche (von Buchholtz, 2000) distinguish his attribution of the symbolic role of animals from that of Freud's, who contended that the imagined animal is representative of unconscious castration fears.

Finally, while Carl Rogers' client-centred model offers a way of considering the therapeutic relationship that departed from traditional psychoanalytic thinking, it is worth taking into account the influence of his humanistic ideas on the oft-cited qualities of companion animals' empathy and unconditional love in studies of pet ownership and animal-assisted therapy (Kruger and Serpell, 2010).

The birth of animal-assisted therapy

Then, in 1961, in an address to the American Psychological Association, Dr. Boris Levenson presented his experiences of the effects of an animal on the therapy of a disturbed child patient (Bachi and Parish-Plass, 2016). Levenson noted, as Freud had done some decades earlier, that the child, who had difficulty communicating, seemed more relaxed and more able to engage in conversation in the presence of an animal, a contention which was met with derision and laughter (Coren, 2013). It was only when Freud's work about his treatment of his patients in the company of his dogs became public that Levenson was able to refer to Freud's writing and had sufficient authority to begin to investigate his observations (ibid).

Subsequently, the research of Beck and Katcher (ibid) demonstrated that physiological changes, in the form of the lowering of sympathetic nervous system activity, occur when humans are in the presence of an animal. While, for some time, pets had casually been included in the psychoanalytic encounter, the attention that Levenson drew to the practice, coupled with the investigations of Beck and Katcher, provided further validation for the inclusion of animals in treatment. This exposure to the practice of including animals in treatment paved the way for the development of animal-assisted therapy (AAT).

Contemporary AAT literature frequently acknowledges loving human-animal relationships, an observation that has become the rationale for the inclusion of animals in a treatment process (Kruger and Serpell, 2010). Many references within the AAT literature explain the human-animal bond by recruiting elements of attachment theory, and Kruger and Serpell (ibid) point out that additionally there are suggestions that pets may be seen as 'transitional objects' (Winnicott, 1951, in Kruger and Serpell, 2010) even in the case of adult patients. Serpell (1999) argues that the advantage of pets over conventional transitional objects is their capacity for responsiveness in alleviating the stress of the initial phases of therapy.

I thus wish to pay tribute here to the oft-cited therapeutic potential of human interaction with companion animals in various clinical settings and the significant work that has been done, attesting to the health benefits (Beck, 2000) of animals, to animals' role in skills training, symptom reduction, and behavioural change, and the psychological and cognitive advantages of AAT (Bachi and Parish-Plass, 2016; Brown, 2004; Kruger and Serpell, 2010).

It is at this juncture that we move to discussing the importance of animals not only as therapeutic in their own right but also to use the language of relational psychotherapy as the third in the room.

Animals in relational psychotherapy

As relational psychoanalysts and psychotherapists, the authors of this book subscribe to the principle that material brought into the clinical space be considered in relation to the contexts of the psychotherapy relationship between client and therapist and of the therapy frame. As the therapeutic relationship and frame will be extensively explored in the subsequent chapters, a brief elaboration follows.

Given that relational psychotherapy is contingent upon engaging with the complexity arising from 'both within and between the analysand's and the analyst's subjective experiences' (Ringstrom, www.iarppaustralia.com.au), relational psychotherapists work with the principle that the quality of the therapeutic relationship is an unmatched influence in facilitating the broadening of relationship and intrapsychic choice. The frame is the therapeutic structure that offers clear and safe boundaries for the unfolding of the therapy relationship and also provides a space for negotiation and for the illumination of aspects of conscious and unconscious material of both patient and therapist (Bass, 2007) that arise within it. As is the case with the therapy relationship, the frame is thus inextricable from the therapy process itself.

Added to this mix, as relational psychoanalysts, the authors recognise and value the occurrence of *enactments* in the clinical space, those 'recurrent patterns of conduct (that) serve to actualize the nuclear configurations of self and object that constitute a person's character' (Atwood and Stolorow, in Ringstrom from www.iarppaustralia.com.au), and the *third*, which Benjamin (2007), in assimilating definitions offered by others, suggests is 'anything one holds in mind that creates another point of reference outside the dyad' (p. 1) and offers 'a quality of mental space' (ibid) in which meaning may be negotiated. In the context of the therapeutic relationship and the frame, the identification of enactments and the third offers the relational psychotherapist and client opportunities for struggling together to find meaning, broadening relational and intrapsychic choice, and potentially for facilitating therapeutic breakthrough.

Against the backdrop of a relational approach, the authors of this volume have been conducting their clinical practices, somewhat unconventionally the literature seems to suggest, in the company of an animal or animals. This apparently unorthodox coalition of a relational psychotherapist, client, and animal has arisen out of a number of situations, whereby the author has found himself or herself in circumstances dictated either by their animals' needs, by the unexpected intrusion into the clinical space of an uninvited animal, by their client's inclination to symbolise the processing and articulation of his/her clinical material through an animal – actual, virtual or imagined – or by the conventions of their own clinical modality. As a consequence of their own experiences of working with a relational sensibility in the presence of an animal, they have found that elements in their practice of contemporary relational psychoanalytic psychotherapy deemed by the literature to be important are amplified and facilitated by the animal presence.

As a result of Jo Frasca's preliminary research for this project, she made some discoveries that we believe are germane to its development. She found that the relative silence within contemporary relational psychoanalytic literature to consider the impact of working in the company of an animal in the clinical environment was not a reflection of the actual occurrence of this practice in the treatment space.

Despite their own experiences, however, some of our authors also note the relative silence in the literature on this topic of working in the presence of an animal within a contemporary relational psychotherapeutic framework. Whether the gap in the literature is due to idiosyncrasy or inhibition, disavowal or taboo, given that a number of relational psychoanalysts do conduct their clinical practice in the presence of animals, the authors of the following chapters propose that definitions of psychoanalytic concepts be broadened to include and legitimise an animal presence in the clinical arena and to offer a foundation for the discussion, comparison, and clinical use within a relational framework of human-animal relationships.

Animals as the third in relational psychotherapy: Exploring theory, frame and practice is thus a constellation of the authors' attentive observations of the impact of the animal (or animals) on their clients, themselves, the therapy relationship and therapeutic processes, their astute subsequent intervention decisions and their thoughtful clinical reflections. The authors demonstrate that the animal as a third in a number of different clinical settings triggers unconscious conflicts, bringing them to life and making them available for analysis in the clinical setting. They argue that it is frequently the very presence of the animal in the treatment arena that provides unique opportunities for the consideration of the individual human psyche as a social-relational construct, for the exploration of underlying intrapsychic and relational processes, and for the development of symbolising and relational capacity.

By elegantly weaving together contemporary psychoanalytically informed theory, compelling case studies, and clinical reflections, the authors give voice to the principles – including relationship, frame, enactments, the third – and practice of working relationally in the presence of an animal. In doing so, they offer contemporary relational psychotherapy both the means and the mandate to incorporate into its thinking, writing, and conversations a feature intrinsic to our relational worlds.

Specifically, in addition to clinical material, Chapters 2–6 offer cogent theoretical considerations of the chemistry between principles of relational psychotherapy and the human-animal bond. Joanne Emmens, in Chapter 2, extends the brief historical overview outlined at the beginning of this chapter by offering a considered literature review covering the appearance of animals in psychoanalytic writing. In this chapter, against the backdrop of the ubiquity of our interspecies relationships with animals, Emmens introduces considerations about the therapeutic value of information gleaned via our object relations with animals, with which she integrates insights about the role played by animals in creating a bridge to aspects of her patients' hitherto disavowed experiences.

While in Chapter 2 Emmens contemplates psychoanalysis's consideration of animals, in Chapter 3 Virginia Rachmani argues that the very pervasiveness of our relationships with animals renders curious the omission from contemporary psychoanalytic literature of an examination of the human-animal bond. By contending that the absence of a viable structure and vocabulary have precluded the clinical exploration of this bond and its potential in relational psychoanalytic psychotherapy, Rachmani convincingly proposes that this oversight may be remediated by extending terminology in order that we might broaden the discussion to include animals as 'relational creatures'.

As an alternative to our tendency either to sentimentalise dogs and their role in the therapeutic process on the one hand or to objectify them on the other, Sean Meggeson in Chapter 4 explores a particular rendering of empathy on the part of animals, and in particular dogs, and demonstrates their capacity for self-other regulation. Through a discussion about inter-species intersubjectivity, specifically in a nonverbal, non-invasive, relational context, Meggeson crafts a compelling argument for the consideration of dogs as legitimate relational agents.

An appreciation of human-animal intersubjectivity also underpins Dor Roitman's explorations in Chapters 5 and 6, wherein he presents an interesting theoretical framework that brings into focus psychoanalytic and neuroscientific findings and relational principles to address the relational processes and multi-level implicit communications between child patients and animals in therapy. By a contemporary elaboration of Freud's thesis mentioned at the beginning of this introduction, Chapter 5 elaborates in further detail upon the features that animals share with humans that make animals 'subjective others' and legitimate partners for relational and interpersonal processes with people in therapy and beyond.

The 'therapy zoo' provides the context for Chapter 6, in which Roitman presents a group-analytic approach. He explores the ways in which group analytic concepts overlap with the principles underpinning the therapy zoo, focusing specifically on group dynamics within animal communities when they are joined by a therapist and a child patient. Using the notion of the Matrix, Roitman comprehensively addresses the multi-dimensional mechanisms, perspectives, and processes that are effective in advancing therapeutic change in such settings.

Staying with the group context, in Chapter 7 David Vincent provides us with some of the fundaments of group analysis and explains the Foulksian group-analytic view of the psychotherapy group boundary, thereby inaugurating a discussion about the complex issues of boundaries and frame that will be further explored in subsequent chapters. In circumstances that diverge from Roitman's in Chapters 5 and 6, where the psychotherapy process is contingent on the presence of animals, Vincent, with a refreshing lightness of touch, adds ballast to the complexities of frame considerations. He shares with us three 'boundary incidents' triggered by uninvited animals that infringed upon the group boundary, precipitating enactments and resulting in the group's emotional and relational progress.

With the introduction of her canine companion into her life, her home, and later on, into her psychotherapy practice, Jo Frasca in Chapter 8 recognises that her dog can be diagnosed as traumatised in accordance with the DSM III classification. She hypothesises that the anxiety her dog displays when they meet parallels that which clients often experience upon meeting a new therapist. Frasca supplements ideas discussed in earlier chapters about the similarities between humans and animals and reflects on how safety and consistency help her traumatised dog to regulate, to improve her social skills, and to develop confidence, all of which contribute to a developmental triumph and all of which is comparable to what clients may experience during the process of psychotherapy. Her description of her dog's trauma history foreshadows an examination in forthcoming chapters about the subjectivity of the dog as one of the factors to be evaluated when intentionally introducing an animal into the therapeutic environment.

In Chapter 9, Gaiana Germani elaborates upon this theme, describing her thoughtful and sometimes fraught process of deciding whether, how, and when to bring her dog, likewise with a history of trauma, into her treatment room. Germani shares with us her concerns about the blurring of boundaries, the impact on her patients of her traumatised dog, and the less-than-encouraging reactions from her colleagues. She pays fine attention to the therapeutic considerations, both practical and psychological, of introducing an animal into the therapy space and once having done so observes how within a 'triad of trauma' her patients made use of her dog to heal.

Frasca, in Chapter 10, continues the conversation about intentionally introducing a dog into the clinical environment. Underpinning such decisions is a cognisance of boundary and frame issues, which Frasca explores, suggesting that bringing the dog into the treatment space may constitute a frame breakage. Frasca describes one consequence of having done so, which was disruptive in the short term. Like Vincent in Chapter 7, she considers how thoughtful attention to the consequences of frame breakages, considered or inadvertent, can gently prise open dialogue to present the clinician with abundant productive information. Frasca introduces us to the Transactional Analysis notion of the *carom* – the opportunity offered to the patient by the presence of, and relationship with, a third object (the dog, in this instance) to express, through itself, the patient's otherwise unspeakable stories and words, in order that the gravity of her internal world may be communicated to the psychotherapist.

Gretchen Heyer, in Chapter 11, continues to scrutinise the somewhat vexed matter of the frame in theory and practice, its advantages and challenges in psychotherapy, and the effects of frame breakages. Heyer's powerful case study explores the impact of animals as unexpected and unwelcome intruders, as was the case with the animals in Vincent's Chapter 7. Heyer addresses another complex area in this chapter. In honouring her patient's historical, socio-political narrative, acknowledging collisions of power, gender, class, and race, and bearing the charged impact of these on their therapeutic engagement, Heyer attentively tackles both the clinical and theoretical dimensions of the intersubjective field that is often overlooked under the guise of assumptions of similarity.

Beth Feldman in Chapter 12 extends the themes introduced in the previous chapters by investigating, through case material, how the influence of her dog is felt in relational psychoanalytic treatment in its most challenging and transformative dimensions. In the context of an authentic patient-analyst relationship and the ability of both patient and analyst to access and share intrapsychic experience, she describes how her dog, as an analytic third, acts as a 'bridge over troubled waters' influencing the clinical space in a way that facilitates the unfolding of unconscious communication, the connection to dissociated feelings and self-states, and the alliance of patient and analyst.

Frasca presents case studies in Chapters 13 and 14 on grief and on fear and anger, respectively, to explain the process of psychotherapy, to demonstrate how the role of her dog in the context of the analytic triad was instrumental in her clients' processing of their material and ultimately how the dog could be seen as significant in her patients' transformation.

In her case study in Chapter 15, Lynn Higgins provides another example of a relational experience whereby one party, the patient, communicates to a second, the analyst, via a safe, non-threatening third – a feature identified by Frasca in Chapter 10, as a *carom*. Higgins describes her patient's relationships with animals – both real and imagined – and the way she makes use of them in her relationship with the analyst. Higgins proposes that this triadic relational system of the patient, analyst, and animal enables her patient's discovery of her words, her growing experience of safety, and the development of her capacity to connect, thereby attesting to the potential of animals whose attributes may support us in finding our words, 'when we have momentarily lost our voice' (Suen, 2013, p. 137).

In our final chapter, Jo Frasca and I recognise the capacity of animals to attune to human emotions, as had Freud in his appreciation of his beloved Jofi (Freud, in Braitman, 2014), Levenson in his justification for including dogs in his treatment of children (Bachi and Parish-Plass, 2016), and some of the authors who have contributed to this book. In this final chapter, we consider the tendency of some animals to comfort patients in distress and in doing so, to mute affect expression. By exploring both the mutative power of affect and the transformative potential of patient-dog engagements we question whether an animal's empathic behaviour, in arresting affect expression, undermines psychotherapy or whether such intuitive action on the part of the animal presents a unique opportunity for understanding the intrapsychic and relational worlds of the patient and thereby facilitates the analytic work.

A fluid interplay of theoretical tenets, contributions from the literature, clinical reflections, and case material in *Animals as the third in relational psychotherapy: Exploring theory, frame and practice* accentuate recurrent themes: animals are seen by human beings as significant subjective others and are treated as legitimate partners for relational and interpersonal processes, as attachment figures, and as transferential objects. Animals in the psychotherapy environment can provide a 'bridge' from the unconscious to the conscious, from the dissociated to the experienced, and from the intrapsychic to the interpersonal. As the third in the treatment arena, the animal is shown to trigger unconscious conflicts, bringing them to life and making them available for analysis in the clinical setting. The authors repeatedly show how deep attention to the human-animal experience in the treatment process can soften the analytic space in ways that encourage progressive communication, understanding of the patient, and the relaxing of defences, leading to the symbolising of relational capacity, therapeutic breakthrough, and intrapsychic change.

Finally, we return to Chiron. In addition to offering an archaic template for the themes that weave through this book, the myth perhaps resides in the collective imaginings of those therapists who work in the presence of an animal. Chiron's story, after all, is a story about a punitive parent manifesting as a feared animal, about early trauma, and being a victim of circumstances. It is a story of the embodiment of early psychological injury, of the repetitive nature, inevitability, and consequences of enactments, of unintentional wounding, and the impact of a third. It is a story about the remedial potential of 'animal empathy', the animal as a bridge – between the world of animals and that of humans, between self-states, between self and other – and about the human-animal bond. It is also a story about despair and hope, disruption and repair, and about compassion, sacrifice, surrender, and choice. The myth reminds us that we – as human animals – are flawed, and that persecution, wounding, and protection occur between us, often inadvertently. Ultimately, the story of Chiron reminds us of the transformative power of the relationship.

Each of the authors who have contributed to this text contends that it is vital to bring into consciousness their – and others' – experiences, observations, and reflections emanating from working psychoanalytically in the presence of an animal and to elaborate upon the discourse of psychotherapy in order that it may be regarded as legitimate to include animals in the therapy space. It is our hope that *Animals as the third in relational psychotherapy: Exploring theory, frame and practice* will extend psychoanalytic and relational principles to create a theoretical framework and language for the consideration of the presence of animals in the clinical space and thus help to authorise the incorporation into the practice of relational psychotherapy the therapeutically eloquent triadic interactions of therapist, client, and animal.

References

Bachi, K. and Parish-Plass, N. (2016) Animal-assisted psychotherapy: A unique relational therapy for children and adolescents. *Sage Journals.* 22(1), pp. 3–8.

Bass, A. (2007) When the frame doesn't fit the picture. *Psychoanalytic Dialogues.* 17(1), pp. 1–27.

Beck, A. M. (2000) The use of animals to benefit humans: Animal-assisted therapy. In A. H. Fine (ed.), *Handbook on Animal-Assisted Therapy: Theoretical Foundations and Guidelines for Practice.* San Diego, CA: Academic Press, pp. 21–40.

Benjamin, J. (2007) Intersubjectivity, Thirdness, and Mutual Recognition. *Presentation to Institute for Contemporary Psychoanalysis,* Los Angeles, CA. icpla. edu > Benjamin-J.-2007-ICP-Presentation-Thirdness-present-send.pdf, Accessed 08/08/19.

Braitman, L. (2014) *Dog complex: Analyzing Freud's relationship with his pets.* https:// www.fastcompany.com/3037493/dog-complex-analyzing-freuds-relationship-with-his-pets, Accessed 12/06/19.

Brown, S. (2004) The human-animal bond and self psychology: Toward a new understanding. *Society and Animals.* 12(1), pp. 67–86.

Coren, S. (2013) How therapy dogs almost never came to exist. *Psychology Today.* https://www.psychologytoday.com/au/blog/canine-corner/201302/how-therapy-dogs-almost-never-came-exist. Accessed 15/06/19.

De Chavez, J. (2015) Dreaming of animals: The animal in Freud's analysis of a phobia in a five-year boy and history of an infantile neurosis. *Rupkatha Journal on Interdisciplinary Studies in Humanities.* 7(3), pp. 38–44. www.rupkatha.com.

Freud, S. (2001) *Totem and Taboo.* London and Routledge: Taylor & Francis Group.

Hannah, B. (2006) *The archetypal symbolism of animals.* https://chironpublications com/shop/archetypal-symbolism-animals/, Accessed 26/06/19.

Jung, C. G. (1995) *Memories, Dreams, Reflections.* London: Fontana Press.

Kruger, K. A. and Serpell, J. A. (2010) Animal-assisted interventions in mental health: Definitions and theoretical foundations. In A. H. Fine (ed.), *Handbook on Animal-Assisted Therapy* (3rd Edition). London: Academic Press, pp. 33–48.

Marinelli, L. and Mayer, A. (2016) The receding animal: Theorizing anxiety and attachment in psychoanalysis from Freud to Imre Hermann. *Science in Context.* 29(1), pp. 55–76.

Molnar, M. (1996) Of dogs and doggerel. *American Imago.* 53(3), pp. 269–280.

Ringstrom, P. Everything you've wanted to know about relational psychoanalysis but were too confused to ask. www.iarppaustralia.com.au > resources > iarpp-resources, Accessed 30/06/19.

Serpell, J. (1999) Animals in children's lives. *Society and Animals.* 7(2), pp. 87–94. https://psycnet.apa.org > record >1999-15443-001, Accessed 20/06/19.

Suen, A. (2013) From animal father to animal mother: A Freudian account of animal maternal ethics. *philoSOPHIA.* 3(2), pp. 121–137. http://muse.jhu.edu/journals/phi/summary/v003/3.2.suen.html, Accessed 15/06/19.

von Buchholtz, J. (2000) Animals and the psyche. *Quarterly News.* www.jungatlanta. com > articles > spring00-animals-and-psyche, Accessed 28/06/2019.

2 Exploration of animal-human relationships in psychoanalytic psychotherapy

Finding pathways to bridge remnant, disowned, or as yet undeveloped parts of self

Joanne Emmens

Introduction

This chapter is concerned with the phenomenon of animal-human relationship and the multitude of ways that these manifest in the lives of ourselves and our patients. Our cross-species relationships with our family pets, memories of animals from our childhood, and associations to animal symbols from stories and mythology are arguably formative experiences in all of our developmental histories. In cases of complex trauma and severe disturbances of the self, this material contains important associations that in a similar fashion to 'dreams' can be harnessed in the service of accessing pathways to parts of self that as a consequence of trauma have become arrested or dissociated from awareness. Psychoanalytic developmental theories within the object relations tradition offer a framework for the exploration of what I have come to register as an elusive territory that necessarily defies any definitive or conclusive definition or pinning down.

Important 'reservoirs for our projections'

Psychoanalysis, from its foundations with Freud, has attributed a special significance to the animal-human bond (Beck and Katcher, 1996; Akhtar and Volkan, 2005). Freud maintained close ties to the Darwinian scientific paradigms of the enlightenment era, emphasizing our similarity and common ancestry to our non-human fellow mammals. In relation to early developmental theory, Freud observed an affinity between pre-verbal children and animals, which he attributed to a readiness to empathically identify with their pet animal companions in a manner that is lost in adult years, observing that '[c]hildren have no scruples over allowing animals to rank as their full equals' (Freud, 1955b, p. 127).

In relation to the real value of animals in his life, Freud is very articulate. His daughter Anna Freud recalls her father's closeness to his dog companions in his later life, and how he openly admitted his gratitude towards their lack of ambivalence. She recalls him saying that 'dogs love their friends and bite their enemies, in contrast to men who are incapable of pure love and must at times mix love and hate in their object relations' (Jacobs, 1994, p. 851).

Freud's friend, fellow psychoanalyst and dog owner, Marie Bonaparte (who gifted to Freud his beloved Chows) wrote a small book in which she describes her relationship with her dog, Topsy, through her pet's diagnosis, treatment, and eventual recovery from cancer. This short book (Bonaparte, 1994) details with deceptive simplicity how Bonaparte's cross-species relationship with Topsy's mortal vulnerability (of which Topsy could not be conscious) allowed her to access her own pre-verbal and wordless fears around mortality, thus capturing her deep sense of attachment to life. In appreciation for Bonaparte's manuscript Freud wrote,

> My Dear Marie
> Just received your card from Athens and your manuscript of the Topsy book. I love it: …..It really explains why one can love an animal like Topsy (or Jo-fi) with such extraordinary intensity; affection without ambivalence, the simplicity of a life free from the almost unbearable conflicts of civilization, the beauty of an existence complete in itself; and yet despite all divergence in the organic development, that feeling of an intimate affinity, of an undisputed solidarity. (Freud, 1960, pp. 434–435)

Freud's interest in and appreciation for working with animal symbols in his work with patients extended beyond an understanding of the impact of direct pets' relationships, as is evidenced in three of his famous case studies 'Rat Man' (1955a), 'Little Hans' (1955a) and 'Wolf Man' (1955c). Each case example serves to illustrate the individually unique way that the patients' fantasies about animals can function as 'reservoirs for [each individual's] projections' (Akhtar and Volkan, 2005, p. xiii) and so, in a similar fashion to dreams, can be worked with to allow access to these previously unconscious territories. Animals (whether as pets, memories, or symbols) therefore can function as conduits, facilitating the process of what Bion (1962) terms 'reverie' (a form of awake dreaming where thoughts begin to symbolize and become thinkable). In essence, the work of psychoanalysis (along with arguably all psychotherapies) is the creative endeavor of facilitating awareness of what has been obscured from our consciousness and so interrupts and distorts our relationship with our internal and external worlds.

The pre-conscious and entrances to 'secret passages' (Bolognini, 2010)

Through the process of this research on the role of animal-human relationships in our object relationships, I have increasingly come up against an intriguing paradox. Many authors (including myself in previous research) found a paucity of psychological research on the topic of animal relationships and even an active dismissing or repudiation (Akhtar and Volkan, 2005; Emmens, 2007). While there is an apparent scarcity of specific literature on this topic, there exists simultaneously an abundance of references to animals and animal symbolism that populate our own and our patients' dreams, reveries and associations, and also potpourri our theoretical papers and constructs. It is as if the topic of animal-human relationships in psychotherapy is hidden in plain view. The nature and complexity of this obscuring are of much interest to me and feel to be an essential and necessary component of this topic. In reference to the complexities of these phenomena in our work, I am reminded of Bolognini's evocative metaphor of our psychological 'cat-flaps' in his book titled 'Secret passages: The theory and technique of interpsychic relations' (Bolognini, 2010). Bolognini uses the symbol of a cat-flap (a small door embedded in the main entrance door to home) to illustrate structurally the functioning of the invariably complex communications between therapist and patient in which projections (from both patient and therapist) manage to come and go (to and fro) unnoticed (just as our cats move freely between indoors and outdoors and sometimes clandestine mice manage to enter the house even while the 'official' door is not kept open by us). Bolognini conjectures that the cat-flap device corresponds to a preconscious mental level and that these interpsychic 'cat-flaps' develop between the patient and therapist couple, providing a useful regulating function. Bolognini observes that over time and with the building of familiarity, the unique conditions of 'analysis "constructs a cat-flap" and coaches the "cat" (the preconscious) to use it' (ibid, p. 67). Throughout his book, Bolognini depicts the infinitely variable ways in which we 'recognize' or even 'catch on the fly' preconscious communications from working with dreams, enactments, and mutual reverie that allow us passage into precious 'secret passages' that become functional by way of us being made aware of them. Bolognini stresses the importance of the unintentional nature of these discoveries which cannot be planned or intentionally set up. In the same way as psychoanalytic 'empathy', Bolognini stresses that these phenomena are events and not reproducible methods or procedures. Rather than a scarcity of research or a repudiation of this topic, perhaps our 'study' of animal-human relationship (which I observe as innately regressive) is facilitative of entry into and along these 'secret passages'. Our relationships with our non-human family members occupy a space that is both real (as our pets are individual and separate beings in their own right) and in Winnicottian terms transitional (as a degree of cross-species imagination and anthropomorphism is inevitable). In my own and my supervisees' clinical experience, I observe that tolerable emotional distance can be fostered when working with a patient's free associations relating to animals (relationships and symbols), which is creatively facilitative of sensitive psychological exploration, allowing security to explore emotions from new perspectives. I am reminded of Ferro's (2013) use of the metaphor 'comfortable oven gloves' in interpreting emotions that are 'still too hot to handle' for the patient. Ferro reminds us of the difficulty in integrating previously 'split-off' emotions without first having the 'space' to contain them.

The adventures of Pinocchio, secret passages and the development of conscience

Within any culture, it seems that animal characters and symbolism in myth, fairy tales, nursery rhymes, popular and classic children's literature, and advertising populate our childhood as well as adult landscapes. The animal characters that populate many of our classic fables stand for symbols of virtue and vice and are used to illustrate dramatic transformations back and forth along these continuums. These nonsensical and fantastical inheritances perhaps contain universal themes functioning as a form of collective cultural 'dreaming'. In this, I am reminded of Bion's use of the metaphor of 'two-way traffic' in his playful suggestion that rather than writing a book on 'the interpretation of dreams', one should instead write a book on 'the interpretation of facts', translating them into dream language – not just as a perverse exercise, but in order to get a 'two-way traffic' (Bion, 1980, p. 29). I suggest that the practice of 'interpreting facts back to dreams' is an essential and principal role of the artist, poet and 'story-teller' within our societies. Such 'translations' offer us narrative and company along many of our developmental pathways towards maturation and the complex and painful process of building our own capacities for 'learning from experience' (Bion, 1962). It is after all necessary to become aware of the cunning charms of 'wolves' (charlatans) and to learn the patience and wisdom of building secure protective houses of bricks rather than giving in to the ease and low cost of straw or sticks. The inherent dangers of remaining stubbornly in folly by refusing to 'learn from experience' (ibid), the consequences of our repetition compulsions (Freud, 1955d) are common and universal dream-like themes of many of these non-sensical tales (or 'translated facts').

For example, the original tales of Pinocchio written in 1883 by Carlo Collodi, contain many dream-like impossibilities and animal characters that allow us to play on the borders of dreaming and waking, of life and death, and reality and unreality. A house cricket functions as the young puppet's external conscience before he has developed a capacity to develop his own internal conscience and capacity for mature object relationships. Pinocchio accidentally kills the cricket with a hammer in a fit of rage when he does not want to be lectured about the importance of being a good and obedient boy, the 'cricket' does not give up on Pinocchio and survives in the form of a ghost cricket to continue his work with the rebellious and defiant Pinocchio. In Winnicottian terms, Pinocchio's journey from object relating to being able to 'use' (and so have a capacity to love and feel loved) his objects was fraught with obstacles and detours yet is ultimately successful due to the dedicated maternal love of the 'fairy'. Perhaps the 'adventures of Pinocchio', from wooden puppet to a real little boy, through many back roads, regressions, refusals and repudiations, parallel many of the psychoanalytic adventures (along secret passageways) that we all journey along with our patients, as we travel towards mature object relations. I believe that a capacity for 'translating facts back to dreams' is fostered in the therapy relationship, facilitating the poetic fluidity of 'two-way traffic' that is strengthening of what Bion calls our alpha functions (our capacity to perceive and to recognize). Bion stresses that 'following psycho-analytic principles, it is clear that the analyst should be alert to the tracking of symptoms in both directions. The problem [he reasons] is not a mind with one track, but a track that is one-way' (Bion, 1980, p. 19).

A patient Melle, described to me her gratitude for what she termed her 'slow, quiet transformation' towards becoming her 'real authentic self' that although not immediately visible on the outside, she considered her greatest life achievement and most significant journey. Melle's 'quiet transformation' seemed to be firstly inspired by her watching documentaries on elephant herds where themes of attachment, loss, mourning and despair slowly became knowable, thus precipitating her own capacity to mourn. Analogous to the tales of Pinocchio, Melle describes her previous life as having been 'wooden' and deadening, where she would alternate between imitative attempts to stay in proximity to her objects and fraught and dangerous periods of protest, anger, depression and despair.

Another patient Will, achieved a beginning capacity for emphatic concern towards another (his partner) and his own early vulnerable dependency, over a four-year psychotherapy in which first the defenses of powerful and dangerous animals were protectively identified with, leading the way to contemplate animals with not so developed defenses and even small (yet survivable) defects and deformities.

In the following paragraphs, I will discuss these two cases in line with our theme of making meaningful use of animal-human relationships (our objects in the room) that find their way into our therapy relationships.

Melle's quiet transformation towards her authentic self

Melle, a 30-year-old woman, suffered a childhood characterized by physical and sexual violence, profound neglect and abandonment. At the beginning of her six-year therapy, Melle's principal concerns revolved around a recent break-up with a man whom she knew to be 'bad for her', physically and emotionally abusive, and who had openly expressed his lack of love or concern for her. Despite knowing that this relationship was unviable, she found that she could not stop herself obsessively thinking about him. She experienced him to 'pop up' in her mind, innumerable times a day, which left her with an unbearable sense of 'not mattering' as a person. These obsessive and at times violently demanding thoughts seemed to fuel Melle's severe depression and suicidal ideation. Melle feared that she would impulsively end her life in a violent fashion without really knowing why.

As an infant, Melle and her siblings were frequently left for days at a time without adequate food and were subject to years of sexual abuse by an older relative. Melle (an intelligent and courageous patient) was quickly able to link her 'felt' sense of the 'pop up ex' (a metaphor that she began to use for this brand of intrusive memory) as belonging to her 'past', where her family would call her a 'nobody'. For Melle, a 'nobody' meant that you were so deficient that you did not reach the category of being a 'person'. A 'nobody', was of no consequence to anybody and worse than being an orphan as any hope of eliciting love or care or of mattering to another 'non-nobody' person was deemed unattainable. It was a grimly definitive category of being that encapsulated a form of felt exile from being a real human being.

Through the process of therapy, Melle increasingly was able to link her habit of forming attachments to emotionally unavailable and/or abusive men who would exploit her, as having origins in her past traumas. She came to realize that the thought of leaving these relationships (or being left) evoked her terror of going back into what she referred to as 'the dark place' of being a 'nobody'. As our work progressed over many years, Melle's experience of deprivation became more apparent and in tiny steps, she started the work of being able to speak about and know her 'past' and to face into the wordless and as yet unthinkable trauma and associated losses of her early life. A definitive turning point occurred when Melle reported to me her interest in elephants and in watching documentaries about elephant herd culture where themes of traumatic poaching, orphaned elephant calves, separation and abandonment of calves, and reunions of mother and calf are movingly depicted. I believe these documentaries functioned as necessary 'oven gloves' (Ferro, 2013) allowing her a form of transitional space (Winnicott, 1971) where she could connect to and contain emotions (Bion, 1962) associated with her own early abandonment and traumatic neglect at a safe and tolerable distance.

Repairing damaged internal objects and faulty equations

Melle was able to imagine the tragedy of an abandoned baby elephant as arguably more painful than that of an orphaned elephant (a mother doesn't choose to be murdered yet a degree of choice, at least, is perceived by an abandoned child). An orphaned elephant (if caught in time) has a possibility of being adopted and loved by a substitute mother (Melle would later recover a protective and sustaining childhood fantasy where she imagined being 'given' to a childless woman who would have treasured the opportunity to be a mother – and in this fantasy, she could imaginatively experience herself as a precious and wanted daughter). The concept of maternal abandonment was before now unknowable as it was unthinkable – to think about this reality was not viable as it would mean the child was actually alone.

The massive defenses employed to shield a child from this unknowable truth is lifesaving yet comes at an enormous psychological cost. As Winnicott's (1971), famous quote 'that there is no such thing as an infant, only mother and infant together' asserts, humans (like elephants) perish without the protection and nurturance of the devoted parent(s).

An abandoned and mistreated child will formulate the equation that it is they that are lacking (defective/bad/faulty) in order to preserve the parent as 'good' and maintain the illusion that if they were to 'fix' themselves, then they would illicit the life-preserving love that in reality is their birthright (Shengold, 1989). I observe that it is a hugely painful and terrifying task to disturb or question this faulty formulation and that it is often clung to like a life raft. For this protective illusion to be maintained it needs to remain in an unquestioned holding pattern of suspended pending. To give up on the 'wait' (albeit an unconscious waiting) for the rejecting object to transform into the much needed protective parent would require facing into and beginning to mourn an as-yet unbearable reality; that those who one most depended on for survival were both absent and destructive towards our being.

Through her attentive watching of the elephant documentaries, Melle was able to conceive of and begin to internalize an early developmental blueprint of the necessary conditions for the development of a self. I believe it was important that the sad reality that not all baby elephants survived such abandonment as a consequence of not all elephant mothers being 'good enough' (Winnicott, 1971) was able to be witnessed and understood for this truth to begin to be mourned. Freud (1957), reminds us that we cannot mourn what we cannot know, and as discussed above, avoiding unbearable and unknowable 'truths' is the modus operandi of our defense system that fuels the creation of our symptoms.

I believe that Melle's viewing of these terrifying and heart-wrenching scenes from a cross-species perspective allowed the necessary 'oven glove' insulation to contemplate the nature of such early relational injuries and to start to contemplate the faulty formulations that preserve an illusion of care (now able to be registered for the first time as an absence). These documentaries illustrated to Melle how an infant elephant calf could not possibly be the cause of their own life-threatening abandonment which opened alternative perspectives to be thought about – such as the mother elephant's own trauma around the threats of poaching, and scarcity of resources. These wonderings led Melle to be able to speculate on the impact of her own family's legacy of intergenerational trauma.

Melle began to recognize an internal sequence of conclusive thoughts that would take her to what she came to refer to as the 'dark box place'. In times of stress, she would experience a 'pop-up' (an image of the unavailable ex-boyfriend/object). She would then feel a familiar equation forming in her mind around the 'question' of whether she was a 'nobody' or a 'somebody'. The now absent and rejecting 'object' (the pop-up ex) would then lend evidence to the 'fact' that she was a 'nobody' and she would feel exiled back to the 'dark box place' which although dismal and depressing, at least offered the relief of the verdict being made and displaced her rage away from her original object (mother) and onto the ex-boyfriend. Later in her therapy, Melle came to recognize that the seductive pull of the 'dark box place' was the illusion that offered a definitive answer – affording her a resting place from the unbearable gamble of hoping for something different as well as protection from journeying out into unknown territory. Melle frequently reminds us both that she won't be stopping anymore at the 'dark box place' as she now realizes the importance of 'feeling [her] own authentic sadness' and of the value of learning to 'trust her loneliness'. Melle observes that although these states are difficult, that they are in the direction of 'moving forward' and most importantly away from 'the dark box place'.

The pufferfish and a 'stupid' deaf cat; finding live habitats for disowned and displaced parts of self

Will, a young man of 25 years, survived a sadistically violent and bleak childhood bouncing between being in the care of his mother (who was addicted to alcohol and drugs), various state care institutions and a series of violent foster homes. A small and cripplingly anxious child Will 'discovered' alcohol in his early teens and tributes his alcoholism with having saved his life. He believed that nobody loved alcohol as much as he and experienced the effects of this as a 'super-power'. However, after a few years, Will began to experience his 'super-power' as waning, and his anxiety returned in the form of psychotic paranoia (that people could see right through him, were accusing him of being homosexual and were planning to rob, sexually exploit and assault him). With alcohol no longer working and feeling in a more and more desperate state, Will increasingly engaged in criminal activities involving escalating vigilante-themed violence.

Identification with the aggressor

Ferenczi (Ferenczi and Dupont, 1933) postulated that the predominant defense available to children who are helpless in the hands of abusing adults is identification with the aggressor. When attachment figures are loving and kind then the child introjects these qualities in a manner that helps strengthen their capacity for independence, care and capacity to look after themselves. When the attachment figures are non-protective, violent, sadistic and terrifying then the child of course introjects these qualities (to an even greater extent) as a defence mechanism against these frightening experiences as indicated by Anna Freud in her example of a girl who counselled her younger brother who was afraid of dogs 'If you be a doggie, the dog won't bite you' (Sandler and Freud, 1985).

A useful early metaphor that we found to symbolize Will's defensive destructive violence and 'prickly' manner, was the 'pufferfish' who has an advanced ability to sense danger and can swell itself up and defend itself with its extremely poisonous spikes. In our therapy, it seemed important to Will that we *together* researched (and were both interested in and appreciative of) this fascinating fish, finding out that it manufactured its own advanced potency of poison by harvesting ingredients from its natural marine environment (so that a pufferfish does not possess any innate poison and if living in a secure tank without enemies will be harmless). I noted a marked shift in our work and notable relaxation in Will after the 'pufferfish' metaphor entered our joint therapy vocabulary. I believed it allowed us the 'oven gloves' to examine both Will's hyper-vigilant defences (his advanced ability to sense danger) as well as his defences of 'harvesting' whatever he could from his hostile and dangerous environment (such as alcohol and violent acting out) to protect himself.

The stupid deaf white cat

As our vocabulary of Will's internal defensive world developed, we were able to increasingly get to know and find language for more vulnerable parts of him that contained a debilitating paranoia and scathing of 'stupidity'. Will read into the gaze of others' that they viewed him as 'stupid' and were calculating how they might exploit or punish him for this. Any perceived criticism (real or imagined) was experienced as confirmation of this paranoia, contributing to a chronic and exhausting sense of living on a perpetual battlefield.

My daughter had at this time adopted a stray white cat which she named Walter. Walter, it turned out, was stone deaf and really not the smartest of cats. He had the habit of knocking objects off shelves and then jumping into the shards (drawing attention to and amplifying the mess he had made). His meow, due to his deafness, was deafeningly loud – so that we would frequently startle. I started to tell Will stories of Walter's exploits so as to introduce a 'character' who was dependent on the care of humans yet whose 'stupidity' was tolerated and even considered endearing. Will, appeared to relish 'stupid' Walter stories and they perhaps offered a tolerable (oven gloves) distance from his own trauma and provided a necessary buffer for his envy. We could speculate on Walter's early life as a stray or abandoned cat, of the possibility of in-breeding (a safe way of exploring his incestuous fears) and ultimately of Walter's innocence and right to be just where he was in his life.

In a session that marked a turning point in our work, Will, seeming to forget himself, burst out for the first time with a spontaneous wish, 'I wish I had a stupid, deaf white cat like Walter'. This was the first time in our work (over a three-year period) that I heard a spontaneous wish being openly verbalized. It was also the first time that I glimpsed an expression of warm vulnerability (a smaller Will). Our work after this session began to increasingly feel easier and that we could for increasing moments of time leave the 'battlefield' (that it felt to me he had forever inhabited) and experience more and more snatches of at least the possibility that the war may end and he could become a citizen (rather than a perpetual soldier) of life.

In small snatches, Will caught moments of feeling able to more comfortably inhabit his own skin. He described 'flashes' of experience where he could look at his partner and see a struggling and separate human (as opposed to his prior scathing conviction that his partner took much pleasure in feeling herself superior to him on account of being further along with the twelve-step program). Will reported an occasion where he noticed his rage subsiding to an unfamiliar feeling of compassion and the beginnings of empathic understanding and noticing. He said, 'maybe this is how she gets to feel good about herself? I noticed when we were at her parents last time, how they – especially her dad – put down everything she says, and she looked sort of sad about it'.

The gamble of recovery – the difficulty of relinquishing protective illusions

Brenman (2006) stresses the essential function of the therapeutic relationship in supporting a patient to arrive at their truth. He observes that a patient will not be able to confront what is intolerable without first having developed a capacity to make use of a supporting object. He writes 'Analysis does not answer historical questions but provides the security to explore them'. Both Melle and Will suffered early and sustained childhood trauma and neglect, which resulted in them being unable to internalise a safe parental object; so their capacity to form relationships with humans at the start of therapy was felt as too dangerous. In both of these very contrasting cases, creative and valuable use was made by 'catching' associations to animal material allowing us access into the realm of intersubjectivity and so understanding of nature and uniquely specific character of their relational injuries. These cases illustrate how working with patients' memories and associations of animals can function firstly to contain (or find lodging) for previously split off 'unthinkable' thoughts and then as a bridge towards developing enough of a sense of safety in our therapeutic relationship to begin to untangle from their traumas and grow towards their authentic (or in Winnicott's (1965) terminology) 'true selves'.

In Alvarez's (1992) brilliant book titled 'Live company' she observes that we cannot help our patients to 're-introject' lost parts of self in a surgical manner as especially in very severe disturbances, 'something may need to grow for the first time' and that this is a 'slow and delicate process' (p. 91). Working with severe disturbance has taught me of the futility of suggesting that a patient has survived their traumatic ordeal until they themselves can find a security to 'discover' this for themselves. Such patients have taught me that the most essential aspect of these joint explorations is that they arise spontaneously within our therapeutic relationships, and in a similar fashion to dreams, are infinitely variable and unable to be pre-determined, prompted, or directed. I believe that allowing ourselves to venture into these imaginative territories of animal-human relating contributes to companionable 'live company' that allows a safe enough emotional distance for the intersubjective relational elements of traumatic material to become first 'dreamable' and then 'knowable', facilitating the essential healing process of mourning. I have learned of the need for consistent negotiation of this 'distance' that carries with it a quality of 'space' that is only able to be determined in the moments of its continual creation. It has been a privilege to travel along these immensely variable 'secret passages' with Melle, Will and many more patients', and to participate in the mutually creative enterprise of these precious discoveries.

References

Akhtar, S., & Volkan, V. (Eds.) (2005) *Animals in the human mind and its sublimations.* London: Karnac.

Alvarez, A. (1992) *Live company. Psychoanalytic psychotherapy with autistic, borderline, deprived and abused children.* London: Routledge.

Beck, A., & Katcher, A. (1996) *Between pets and people: The importance of animal companionship.* West Lafayette, IN: Purdue University Press.

Bion, W. (1962) *Learning from experience.* London: Karnac Books.

Bion, W. (1980) *Bion in New York and São Paulo.* London: Karnac Books.

Bolognini, S. (2010) *Secret passages. The theory and technique of interpsychic relations.* London: Routledge.

Bonaparte, M. (1994) *Topsy: The story of a golden-haired chow.* New York: Bunswick and Transaction Publishers.

Brenman, E. (2006) *Recovery of the lost good object.* New York: Routledge.

Collodi, C. (1883) *Pinocchio.* New York: Open Road Integrated Media.

Emmens, J. (2007) *The animal-human bond in the psychotherapy relationship: As a bridge towards enhanced relational capability.* A dissertation submitted to Auckland University of Technology in partial fulfilment of the degree of Master of Health Science in Psychotherapy.

Ferenczi, S., & Dupont, J. (Eds.) (1933) *The clinical diary of Sandor Ferenczi.* Cambridge, MA: Harvard University Press.

Ferro, A. (2013) *Supervision in psychoanalysis; the São Paulo seminars.* London: Routledge.

Freud, S. (1955a) Two cases histories ('Little Hans' and the 'Rat Man'). In *The standard edition of the complete psychological works of Sigmund Freud, Volume 10 (1909),* J. Strachey (ed). London: Hogarth Press, pp. 3–251.

Freud, S. (1955b) Totem and taboo and other works. In *The standard edition of the complete psychological works of Sigmund Freud, Volume 13 (1913–1914),* J. Strachey (ed). London: Hogarth Press, pp. 1–162.

Freud, S. (1955c) An infantile neurosis and other works. In *The standard edition of the complete psychological works of Sigmund Freud, Volume 17 (1917–1919),* J. Strachey (ed). London: Hogarth Press, pp. 3–124.

Freud, S. (1955d) Beyond the pleasure principle. In *The standard edition of the complete psychological works of Sigmund Freud, Volume 18 (1920–1922),* J. Strachey (ed). London: Hogarth Press. pp. 1–134.

Freud, S. (1957) Mourning and melancholia: On the history of the psycho-analytic movement, papers on metapsychology and other works. In *The standard edition of the complete psychological works of Sigmund Freud, Volume 14 (1914–1916)*, J. Strachey (ed). London: Hogarth Press The Hogarth Press, pp. 237–259.

Freud, S. (1960) *The letters of Sigmund Freud*. New York: Basic Books.

Jacobs, A. (1994) Freud and the interpretation of the wolf-man dream: A dog story? *Contemporary Psychoanalysis*, 30(4): 845–854.

Sandler, J., & Freud, A. (1985) *The analysis of defense: The ego and the mechanisms of defence revisited*. New York: International Universities Press.

Shengold, L. (1989) *Soul murder: The effects of childhood abuse and deprivation*. New Haven, CT: Yale University Press.

Winnicott, D. (1965) *The maturational processes and the facilitating environment: Studies in the theory of emotional development*. The International Psycho-Analytical Library, 64, pp. 1–276. London: The Hogarth Press and the Institute of Psycho-Analysis.

Winnicott, D. (1971) *Playing and reality*. New York: Brunner-Routledge.

3 Relational creatures

The selfobject functions of dogs in psychoanalytic theory and practice

Virginia Rachmani

I am because my little dog knows me.
Gertrude Stein (In Curnutt, 1999, p. 291)

The canine-human bond has long been a strong, interspecies tie in the English-speaking world. And the number of households in which people currently share their life with a dog continues to swell; over eighty-seven million such families reside in the United States alone (American Pet Products Association, 2019–2020).

More than in the past, our psychotherapy offices seem to echo with narratives of patients' relations with furry companions that sometimes underscore their unmet psychic needs with other humans. Clinicians may also share their homes or professional offices with dogs, presenting transferential and countertransferential opportunities or quandaries.

It seems an oversight then that throughout the history of psychoanalysis, no formal theory or even serious discussion of this important non-human interconnection has been attempted. Dogs have instead been impounded in the totems, amulets, metaphors and symbols of our Freudian and Jungian legacies. Perhaps, until the advent of the relational turn, writing about our intimate, interspecies relationships may have been deemed too sentimental, unscientific or prosaic. Many major theorists have privately shared their personal attachments to their dogs but have not written psychoanalytically about these important relationships – leaving us few words with which to discuss the human-canine bond.

As a starting point, I begin by discussing Winnicott's theory of *transitional objects and phenomena* and Kohut's development of *selfobject function*, two important tenets of relational theory. My thinking is augmented by new findings about dogs' domestication, reflections on human-canine mergers in mythology and fetishisms, *canine companioning,* anthropomorphism, unconditional love, and with illustrative cases from among my patients.

Although, we cannot overlook the projections many people place on their pets, nor the psychotic elements that exist for others (see Akhtar and Volkan, 2005), our companion dogs, I suggest, can primarily be understood as the templates for unique, intersubjective and potentially structure-building experiences. I use the term *relational creature*, as a descriptive for those dogs that live closely with people. I also suggest that we adjust what Aron (1996) entitled 'a meeting of minds' for inter-human communications, to *a meeting of affects* to indicate the close, implicit interplay between our species.

Domestication

Serious scientific examination of our remarkable history with dogs begins at the ebbing of the nineteenth century, when Darwin (1998) publishes *The Expression of the Emotions in Man and Animals* in 1872, a year after his *Descent of Man* unsettled the scientific and religious sensibilities of Western society. Anyone living with dogs can easily recognize their facial expressions from Darwin's drawings in this text. He reasons that their barking 'serves to express their various emotions and desires ...having been acquired through domestication...and inherited in different degrees by different breeds... owing to dogs having long lived in strict association with so loquacious an animal as man' (ibid, p. 352).

'Because humans, in effect, created dogs through domestication, the canine mind reflects back to us how we see ourselves through the eyes, ears, and noses of another species' (Berns, Brooks and Spivak, 2012, p. 4). According to mitochondrial DNA tests, 'the oldest uncontested, Palaeolithic remains' (Botiqué, Song and Scheu, 2017, p. 1) of dogs and humans cohabitating are found in Germany as long as at least 20,000 years ago. These dogs were used by man for various tasks such as hunting or guarding, but it was not until the Victorian era in England that dogs were raised for express purposes like work or companionship, creating the standardized breeds we know today (Worboys, Strange and Pemberton, 2018) and elevating the potential for satisfying connections between dogs and diverse groups of people – such as police officers or the disabled.

Early psychologist, Francis Galton (in Heiman, 1956, p. 569) soon supports Darwin's views, writing that dogs have 'an inborn liking for man' and that 'dogs and people...are intelligible to each other...Every whine or bark of the dog, each of his fawning, savage or timorous movements is the exact counterpart of what would have been man's behaviour, had he felt similar emotions'. Discussing Heiman's paper, Linn (in Searles, 1960) makes a leap into interspecies intersubjectivity when he asserts that 'dogs are capable of participating in emotional relationships with humans that seem almost as complicated bilaterally' (p. 17). We may soon have biological proof about this correlation: neuroscientists at Emory University have recently trained dogs to lie still, unrestrained, during fMRI screenings, and compared their reactions to various emotive stimuli with those of human beings. Similar response patterns are found between them, particularly in their respective, dopamine-sensitive caudate nuclei (Berns, Brooks and Spivak, 2012).

Psychoanalytic theory

Warwick University's John Fletcher (2007, p. 1242) traces three world-changing alterations of human narcissism first cited by Freud in 1917 'Copernicus's decentring of the Earth in relationship to other planets'; Darwin's theory of evolution that decentres humans from the animal world, and Freud's 'decentring of the individual to himself for with the discovery of the unconscious, the ego was no longer master in its own house' (pp. 1242–1243). Freud encapsulates mankind's predicament: we are each along the spectrum of narcissism, the final blow being the most basic for every psychotherapeutic investigation. We have not shed our understanding of the second, I argue – our relationship with other animals.

As an example of early unconscious decentring, Winnicott's (1971) concept of the transitional object presupposes that exciting objects, such as I propose family pets, might be used as these way-stations between inner and outer reality – not only with the proverbial stuffed animals. They can act as 'soothers' (p. 7), as well as satisfying Winnicott's requirement that the objects 'must seem to move, or to have texture, or to do something that seems to show it has a vitality or reality of its own' (p. 6). After being decathected, the maturing child reinvests some of his narcissistic energy back onto his parents or other adults. She can also exchange, trade, or transfer them onto other non-human environments and can retain narcissistic ties with her relational creature, enjoying a sense of mastery and satisfying relationships with animals, who provide the experience of 'instrumental empathy' (Ulman and Paul, 2006, p. 47). When domestic animals are enjoyed transitionally, I speculate that they prepare the stage for later engagement and enjoyment. I watched our newly walking, year-old son chase our cat squealing protowords, 'at', 'at', before napping with his stuffed cat, 'Kit', another transitional object-word. His delight and ease with animals first lodged in this 'intermediate area of experience' (Winnicott, 1971, p. 2) during toddlerhood remains today. But when unhappy experiences with a pet occur early on, I believe, anxieties can later be activated.

Neurobiology sets the stage for transitional thought. Schore (2003) describes how at about age three, the left hemisphere takes control over the earlier developing, emotional, right brain, and the child's conscious mind – with its symbolising capacity – commences development. Between the age of two and a half and three years, however, the right brain remains dominant as the left begins 'its growth spurt' (p. 244), as does the corpus callosum, both of which may enable an intermingling of the two sources of knowledge – feeling and language.

Although Kohut's (1971) *The Analysis of the Self* seeks to show how narcissistic individuals can be treated by examining their *archaic selfobjects* – or those which became traumatically embedded due to early parental failures. His conception of *selfobjects* quickly extends Winnicott's thinking to people without narcissistic personality disorders: they are objects that are 'used in the service of the self and the maintenance of its instinctual investment, or

[are] objects which are themselves experienced as part of the self'; they are not necessarily people but can be "non-human" (Kohut, 1977, pp. 56–57)'. Under ordinary circumstances, these functions are first served by the parents who supply *mirroring,* or 'I am perfect and you admire me' and relationships with *idealizable* figures 'you are perfect and I admire you' (Goldberg and Mitchell, 2000). According to intersubjectivists, Stolorow and Brandchaft (1987), 'they designate a class of psychological *functions* (authors' italics) pertaining to the maintenance, restoration and transformation of self-experience' (p. 241), by means of affect integration. Gertrude Stein's 'little dogs' are prime examples of selfobjects: her understanding illustrates how she counterbalances her growing fame with her self-definition in order to feel psychologically cohesive.

Being both interpersonal and intrapsychic, selfobjects argue against the dominance of drive theory and are embedded in the evolution of relational theory by notable luminaries as Jessica Benjamin, Lew Aron, Donnel Stern and Phillip Bromberg, who have developed theories about the third, self-states, enactment, trauma and dissociation in innumerable books and papers.

Twinship selfobjects (sometimes called *alterego selfobjects* by Kohut, 1971, 1977, 1980), were added as a third selfobject category by Kohut; they provide the satisfaction usually attributed to our participation with other people, where we achieve the sense of being 'a human among humans' (1984, p. 200). With personally important animals, many people feel like *a creature among creatures* – and thus gain entrance to the larger world of beings. Although *twinship* and *alter ego selfobjects* are essentially alike, Detrick (1986) clarifies, they operate somewhat differently. The central function of *twinship* is the acquisition of skills, like opportunities to learn caring, nurturing, the containment of aggressive affects and a heightened awareness of the external world. When dogs provide an *alterego selfobject* experiences, they might proffer gratifying occurrences, like meeting other dog lovers at a park with implicit socialization opportunities.

Brothers (1993) amplifies Detrick's conception of the alterego selfobject asserting that it represents the 'hidden or disavowed aspects' (p. 192) of patients and enables them to find self-cohesion. Virginia Woolf (1933) illustrates Brothers' thinking when writing about the poet Elizabeth Browning's relationship with her titular dog *Flush*. Browning, Woolf believes, admires Flush's disobedience and self-serving ways, since she, a Victorian-era woman, must conform to her society's gender restrictions. Woolf imagines Browning thinking, 'There was an alikeness between them. As they gazed at each other each felt: Here am I – and each felt: But how different. Could it be that each completed what was dormant in the other?' (ibid, p. 31).

Psychoanalysts' dogs

Despite Freud's continual confrontation with his unconscious, his enthusiasm for Darwin's work and his love for his own dogs during the last two decades of his life, he has not included his personal feelings for his animals as part of either his metapsychology or in memoir. Freud 'dog-sits' for his daughter Anna's Alsatian, Wolf, and grows so enamoured of him that his former analysand, Dorothy Burlingham, gives him his first Chow, Lin Yug (Gay, 1988). Freud is later 'inseparable' from another Chow, Jo-Fi, who 'would sit quietly at the foot of the couch during the analytic hour' (ibid, p. 540).

Psychoanalyst Marie Bonaparte, a close friend of Freud's, is the rare exception among his early adherents when writing about her own relationship with her dog, 'Topsy'. In the foreword to Bonaparte's poignant memoir about her Chow's cancer treatment, Anna Freud writes, 'what Freud valued in his dogs was their 'gracefulness, devotion and fidelity' (Freud, 1995, p. 301).

Praising their respective Chows in his letters to Bonaparte, Freud says that dogs'

> simplicity... [is] free from the unbearable conflict with civilization, the beauty of existence complete in itself. And in spite of the alien nature of its organic development a feeling of intimate relationship – an undeniable sense of belonging together – exists between us. When stroking Jo-Fi, I have often caught myself humming a melody, which, though quite unmusical, I could recognize as the aria from Don Giovanni (Jones, 1957, pp. 225–226).

When describing the human-canine bond developmentally, Freud (1946) foreshadows Kohut's *twinship selfobject transference*: 'The child unhesitatingly attributes full equality to animals; he probably feels himself more closely related to the animal than to the...adult' (p. 164). Author Margaret Rawlings's young protagonist, Jody, expresses this idea in her Pulitzer Prize-winning novel *The Yearling* (1966), when with no friends near his home in the Depression-era Florida Everglades, Jody tells his mother about his unusual relational creature Flag, a fawn, saying 'He don't seem like a creetur to me, Ma. He seems jest like another boy' (p. 227).

Anna Freud regards psychoanalysis as her 'twin' because she was born in 1895, the year to which her father attributes his discovery of the psychological relevance of dreams (Young-Bruehl, 1988); she later considers Wolf her twin, then Dorothy Burlingham claims this title until her death when Anna says her new Chow puppy Jo-Fi, named after her father's favourite, inherits this role (ibid, p. 444). Through her dogs, Anna appears to complete a developmental quest for her own deeper twinship selfobject relationship with her father. In the *Personal Tributes* (Bulletin of the Anna Freud Centre, 1983) to Anna after her death, her dogs are frequently recalled, particularly Jo-Fi, whom Lampl-de Groot (ibid, p. 55) says is 'a little lion...beautiful but wild'. Alice Colonna (ibid, p. 99) remarks that 'Despite the difficulties of chewed legs, mangled furniture and escapades [Anna] continued to love Jo-Fi, and this may have contributed to her liveliness, even after she became very ill'. Anna disregards these relationships in her own theoretical work.

Jung (1989) speaks of his own childhood affinity for all 'warm-blooded' animals. Dogs are 'dear and faithful, unchanging and trustworthy' he says (pp. 66–67). These words echo his ambivalence in his description of his mother, who has a 'hearty animal warmth and is companionable and pleasant...and a ready listener...But at night, [she] seemed uncanny...like a priestess in a bear's cave...archaic and ruthless' (Jung, 2011, p. 48).

Kohut relishes his ritual, nightly walks with his dog Tovey, according to his biographer (Strozier, 2001, p. 108). Tovey even 'writes' to Anna's dog Coco, following Anna's 1966 visit with Kohut in Chicago. Here, he reveals the pervasiveness of our culture's often light-hearted anthropomorphism. And yet, Kohut never lives long enough to develop a theory to include his relationship with his beloved dog.

Today's theorists feel increasingly comfortable with self-disclosures about their feelings for their dogs. Among the most moving papers is Marcus's (2007) description of the dynamics – based on the work of the philosopher, Emmanuel Levinas – of his love for 'Harry', a rescued Cocker Spaniel.

Merger – between dogs and humans

Human imagination has created mergers between animals and humans for centuries. Merger-hungry societies have drawn on myth or religion as people sought to comprehend the unknowable and to alleviate anxiety. Needs for strength, protection or the avoidance of fear-inducing others encourage the belief in human-animal mergers or chimeras. Dogs are mated in myth with demigods and with humans to produce 'dogmen' according to Atsma (2000–2019), who demonstrates that Hesiod writes of Cynocephili, half dog and half man, born of relations between Gaia, the Earth and Zeus's son Epaphos. Variations of this theme continue among later writers; in 1911 Greece, Brill (1943) tells of hearing a commonly known myth of the Kuno-Andros, the product of an isolated woman having sex with her dog.

Freud, Jung believes, is oblivious to his own mother fixation when he adopts the Oedipus story as the central metaphor of drive theory (in Beebe, 1997), and Jung characterises mothers as 'double beings'. He asserts that Freud fails to see the powerful example of the mythological Sphinx – which is part woman and part dog – calling it 'a fear animal' and a 'mother derivative' (ibid, p. 5).

Undaunted, Freud (1961) embeds his description of the fetish within the oedipal story and his theory of sexuality. To summarise, the little boy learns that his mother has no penis and then fears his own castration by his father. He substitutes an object for her missing penis, and under intense castration anxiety over his own sexuality, uses this fetish object symbolically. This interplay of absence and presence is central to the understanding of the defence of *disavowal*, which Freud introduces within his explanation of fetishism, making it paradoxically 'both a defeat and a victory' (Bass, 1991, p. 309).

Fetishes can be understood as mergers between a person and any object representing the maternal phallus. Winnicott (1971) urges that the word fetish be limited to the 'normal' and

> universal … persistence of a specific object or type of object …linked with the delusion of a maternal phallus, and it should be used solely to describe the infant's experience in the transitional field, although it can develop as an adult fetish if the illusion persists (p. 9).

Freud limits his use of the fetish to males but Greenacre (1955) suggests the possibility of a female fetishist. Later (1969), she stipulates that whether or not a mother has been 'good enough', there is some kind of problematic object relationship in fetishism. It is often an acute experience of seeing the mother's injury, she asserts, and is connected to a 'female body part, another child, or a pet' (ibid, p. 160); Richards (1993) agrees. While discussing her female patient population, she includes animals as one fetish choice used during masturbation. Freud (1962) limits his ideas regarding animals as sexual object choices for limited access to appropriate objects on farms.

Narcissistically disordered individuals (Kohut, 1971) often form selfobject mergers (an extremely primitive form of the mirroring need) with their analysts, using the clinician as a fetish object. Wolf (1988) repositions merger more prominently as another part of the selfobject family. Patients, Wolf asserts, craving a *merger selfobject*, demand the experience of a complete fusion with the mirroring selfobject or hegemony over an idealised selfobject. 'Merger hungry personalities…need to control their selfobjects because they use them in lieu of self structure' (ibid, p. 74); in the transference, the patient needs the analyst to 'be totally subject to [his] initiative' (ibid, p. 124).

Merger hunger patients and animal fetishists can coexist, as illustrated next.

Evie

Baker (1984) reports the case of a young man who masturbates against his dog and at other times 'growled' and 'snarled' at Baker in sessions, reminding me of Evie. Her small dog, Leonardo, serves multiple selfobject functions – as a sole companion, confidant and fetish. Evie's complex interactions with Leonardo offer an opportunity to look at selfobject splitting, a reminder that as with any object choice, there can be a range of functions.

At age thirty-two, Evie has never had an intimate, human relationship. She grudgingly attended thrice-weekly sessions with me for just over three years during an early phase of my analytic training, ending when I could no longer accept her low fee.

Evie is very tall and grossly obese – with the unfinished facial appearance of a toddler. Her flat affect, demeaning attitude and pungent body odour are off-putting to me countertransferentially, the latter of which earns her the label, 'the smelly lady' by denizens of the clinic. She is also rageful, refusing to consider any mutuality between us.

Evie outlines her lonely, fantasy-driven childhood and insufficient, parental attunement; television, she says, particularly old sitcom characters, provide her with access, albeit superficially, to a peer group experience; she recites whole episodes from 'Friends' and 'Charmed', within which she considers herself 'the fourth witch'. Growing up in a lower-middle-income, immigrant family, Evie blames her mother's early death and her father beating her for this object wasteland, which accounts for her feeling entitled to avoid employment. Her narcissistic rage is directed toward any authority figure – and now me.

Sleeping most of the day, Evie survives on fast food supplemented by Hershey bars. She lives with her aging dog, Leonardo, a male, mixed breed, whom she says, looks up at her admiringly, confirming that she is the focus of his life – or to paraphrase Kohut 'the gleam in the dog's eye'– which indicates Leonardo's mirroring and twinship availability, so that he is essential to her wellbeing. She showers him with praise about his appearance and talents and tells me that Leonardo is better than a man: 'He chose me; just wandered up to me near my train stop and followed me home'. When I ask her if she had looked for his owner, she shrugs and says gleefully, 'He's all mine now'.

Evie's messy apartment, she says, is piled high with old books about witchcraft and the occult, which seem to help fortify Evie's efforts to feel as if she knows more than other people – particularly her therapist. She currently rents a basement apartment in a neighbour's house in the same New Jersey suburb where she grew up. Evie cites specific dates and places as she relates her history, acquainting me with her childhood landscape and documenting when and where important events occurred; She grounds herself in the facts and rigorously limits her answers during my detailed inquiry – as if she has been captured by terrorists and gives only her name, rank and serial number.

When Evie is two, her mother dies in childbirth delivering her sister Leona, who then becomes 'Pop's obsession; I was basically told to get lost. I was a kid and couldn't leave, so I just stayed in my room and watched the old black and white TV', Evie moans. But Leona proves to be compensatory. Evie enlists the little girl as her ally, teaching her how to shoplift from nearby stores. 'I could set her up, get Dad to catch her with some toy in her pocket, and yell at her. He liked her anyway. But Leo liked me best', Evie boasts. 'We were inseparable, even taking baths together and having sleepovers in each other's beds'. 'Leo'? I ask, confused.

Oh, that's my sister's nickname. Leo was what I called her when we were alone. She liked it better than Leona. Stupid name. I would just run my hand along her little arm with its blond fuzz, and she would hum.

When Evie and Leona are eight and six respectively, living in the 'horrible Meadowbrook house', their father finds the girls in the bathroom, their underpants on the floor and Evie's hand on Leona's crotch. 'Pop freaks out', Evie chortles, but the incident triggers her numerous beatings.

> I promised myself that I'd get back at him if it was the last thing I ever do. You know what he said, he called me a 'lezzie', said I liked girls not boys, so I needed payback and tried to make him think he was losing his mind.

'How'? I ask.

> Just stuff like pouring salt into the sugar bowl. What'ya think I could do, use arsenic? I was just a kid. He finally died when I was in high school, and we were sent to live with his sister. Good riddance.

Although the sisters remain like 'Siamese twins' into early adolescence, Evie feels that they had been banished from the Garden of Eden – because now Leona understood that what they had been doing was 'dirty'. 'Then,' Evie grimaces, 'Leo leaves home for college and marries a jerk she meets there; I went to a local college. My sister teaches fifth grade now and has two brats of her own'. 'What kind of relationship do you have with Leona now?' I inquire. 'Her husband's an A-hole. That enough for you, doc?' Leona's abandonment of Evie leaves her with a significant object void – a twinship derailed – that she now fills with Leonardo, her dog. When I wonder again about her choice of the same nickname, Leo, for both her dog and her sister, Evie bristles but acts surprised before she quickly reverts to her characteristic ire at my drawing attention to her blatant verbal connection between her most important selfobjects.

Working with Evie does encourage her ongoing font of dream images, past and present; she brings in multiple journals she had written as an adolescent when she was 'dragged to therapy', Evie scowls. Her school had told her father that they thought she was 'troubled'. 'The psychiatrist just wanted me to talk about my mother. I don't even remember her.' I ask Evie, 'what's that like not remembering your mother?' Evie shrugs indignantly.

Any request for her dream associations also causes Evie to crinkle her nose and growl at me like Baker's aforementioned patient. She barks: 'I just told you a dream story. That's all there is. You tell me, you're the fucking analyst'. Her ability to recall details in dreams feels embroidered as if she has reviewed them many times so that they sound more like stories than dreams. As such, they remain narcissistic fantasies that serve the purpose of excluding intrusions of an unempathic world. Leaving me outside of these soliloquies concretizes Evie's illusory world of which she maintains magical control.

Evie's dreams primarily involve stray dogs and cats, or Leonardo, who takes on a supernatural aura with powers that defy gravity: he might shoot into outer space or dive deep into the Hudson River for hidden treasure.

A dream typically plays out as 'I see Leonardo looking up at the North Star, and he tells me that he is going there to visit our grandparents. And then, switching the dog's genders back and forth, she says, 'I tell her that she can't go tonight because she has the flu. We're in the old Meadowbrook house, so I really start to worry. Then she just disappears, popping up on the moon. It's huge, full, like a Hollywood moon. Like that old Cher film, 'Moonstruck', where her grandfather walks his pack of dogs to the East River, and they howl at it. Then everything turns dark; the moon goes out like a light'. Evie's eyes are wide with childlike fright. 'I take a running jump, trying to grab Leo, but he's gone'.

Evie's association with her idealized, alterego superdog can be seen as a needed identification, for he had 'chosen her'. She is special. But at the same time, Evie feels unsafe in the dream when Leonardo leaves home without her like Leona has done. The moon even leaves her alone in the dark – in the house where her father discovered the girls' incestuous proclivities that had initiated Evie's beatings – a loss of twinship opportunities and accounting for decided developmental disruptions. Evie cannot hold onto Leona/Leonardo, nor does she have an opportunity for having more mature sexual satisfaction.

In our third year together, Evie's dreams that she is the fourth witch on 'Charmed', and she begins to include men.

> Last night, Leo and I were touring the Milky Way. Cool, huh? I was free to do whatever I wanted. I see this hot guy, and he starts to take off my clothes. But then I find out that he's really a zombie. I'm scared shitless and go home. Leo's relieved too, but he has been hurt; he has a little mark on the middle of his forehead.

'How did Leonardo get the mark'? I wonder to her. She ignores the question. I add, 'You asked me about my birthmark a few weeks ago', I continue. Evie never mentions my presence in her myriad dreams. Am I perhaps the scary zombie? Am I hurt like Leo? Evie is silent as I tap the birthmark on my forehead. She shrugs, perhaps embarrassed by what I feel is our growing intimacy. In the transference, does Evie see me as a new relational creature, 'a new kind of animal instead of a new object' (Akhtar and Brown, 2005, p. 30).

Leonardo dies during Evie's last few months of our work together. For the first time, she calls me, weeping, and allows me to express my sadness for her loss. Her dreams become littered with images of Leonardo, of Leona, and of flying dogs. She states matter-of-factly that she wants to tell me a 'secret' that feels to me like a reward amid her newfound candour. Evie says that she has surreptitiously frozen Leonardo in her landlord's old freezer in her basement apartment. 'He said I could use it for stuff'. Then, Evie confides tentatively that she misses Leonardo late at night when she masturbates, the time when she would stroke the dog and fantasise. 'He wants me to', she adds. This sexually addictive behaviour seems like a revival of Evie's narcissistic fantasies while stroking little Leona's arm for comfort and as a residue of her childhood need for affect regulation in a chaotic home. Leonardo the dog, like Leona, is dutifully transitional, 'soft, smelly, furry, pliable, warm, and concretely available' (Tolpin, 1971, p. 331).

Evie soon reports, more defiantly, that she is spending nights examining computer pornography, 'there's stuff for girls, too', she tells me knowingly. But Evie acknowledges that she feels empty and depleted afterward. I notice how she has begun to lose weight due to her refraining from binging at night. These nocturnal forays are futile attempts to resurrect a twinship and her traumatic losses of her mother and Leona/Leonardo in succession. But her resulting vulnerability to lifelong loneliness does contain, I feel, a 'forward edge' (Tolpin, 2007), a plea for more human interaction, indicative of our budding relationship and the hot guy. When I tell her what I think, she retorts, 'maybe'. It is Evie's first 'maybe' in our three years together.

I suddenly realize how Evie no longer leads with her repellent body odour, allowing me to resurrect questions about her phobic responses to bathing, and her enormous weight gain after Leona left for college. She explains, 'Pop always stipulated, only one bath a week', she starts to sob quietly, looking heartbroken.

Evie's animal dreams fall off precipitously; although she remarks that she misses 'seeing' Leonardo, she likes her dreams about 'boys'. A few weeks before Evie and I terminate our work, she makes a surprising announcement: 'I made out with that guy who was eyeing me at Mass'. (Evie has resumed attending her childhood church.) 'He kissed me, and I kissed him back. No sex though. I thought nobody would ever kiss me again.' Evie and I sit in silence, aware of the import of our closeness and of her newly found romantic stirrings.

Our ongoing transference-countertransference deadlock is broken in this third clinical year as mutuality and trust enter our sessions, decreasing frequent enactments and expanding Evie's opportunity for growth, as seen in her newfound dating. Albeit initially unnerving to her, the kissing holds the promise of a more mature sexual self-states to emerge and for Evie's greater self-cohesion. Deficits like an absent mother figure, Tolpin (1971) purports, create a lack of the secure base a caregiver provides and the search for a *transitional selfobject* seeks to replace the missing mother. Leona, then Leonardo, became *transitional selfobjects* supplying integral mirroring opportunities, but both not only become twinship selfobjects but are fetishized. Left alone, Evie could not grow into adolescence, seemingly trapped in childhood forever. Leonardo's death, however, sets into motion Evie's risking greater human contact with me and with her emergence into an expanded social setting, which relieves her shame over her fetishistic behaviour and encourages her emotional growth. As we part, I realize how sorry I feel to never hear about Evie's next achievements.

Canine companioning

The overused trope, *'man's best friend'*, encompasses camaraderie rather than merger; it is instead a kind of twinship selfobject experience with an idealizable canine. Rudyard Kipling's short story classic, 'Garm – a hostage' is an example, depicting a hardened soldier's philosophically astute dogs, Garm and Vixen, who, he says, are 'two of the happiest "people" in all the world' (in Teasdale, 2010, p. 60). These relationships may resemble, or act as surrogates for, the unique feeling of closeness with fellow humans that Robert Grossmark (2018) describes in his innovative treatise on *'therapeutic companioning'*.

Grossmark's (2018) conception of *companioning,* influenced by Kohut, the Boston Change Study Group, the Balints, and particularly Stern's unformulated experience and neo-Bionian field theory, is a new register of thirdness within the traditional relational matrix and illustrates his insightful psychoanalytic meditation on working with dissociative, frustrating or baffling patients. It is largely dependent upon the difficulty and its overcoming in analyses of borderline symptomology, with insights gleaned from the contemporary interest in unrepresentational states. In companioning, the clinician accompanies the patient in a 'self-effacing manner into the worlds of inchoate pain, emptiness, darkness and illusion', instead riding a 'flow of enactive engagement' (p. 40) in search of new meanings as the analytic couple surrenders to places unknown and unforeseen. The analyst remains 'unobtrusive and yet deeply involved,' says Grossmark (ibid, p. 40), as he swims the emergent field.

Canine companioning is instead about being 'man's best friend'. It only shares with psychoanalytic *companioning* the 'flow of enactive engagement', which can comfort traumatic losses unable to be reached by traditional technique. But it remains devoid of Grossmark's analytic thought, intent or intellectual rigour.

Because an adult patient's childhood history with animals, whether with pets, strays or even or idealizable, television canines like Lassie, is embedded in the context of her family and cultural milieu, making inquiry into her child-animal relationships can reap substantial clinical information that better explains her affective states than does memory per se. An example is my former patient, Eric, who tells me why he rescues and rehabilitates pit bulls. When he is twelve, Eric brings home an abandoned puppy; his father snatches the clumsily tied rope leash, goes to a nearby wood and shoots the dog. The boy, now a man, remains inconsolable and fantasises about retaliation with his now-deceased father. Meanwhile, he struggles with long-time drug abuse, clinging to his fantasy of each new dog as a panacea. Initially uncomfortable with Eric's violent past, I am mollified by our mutual comfort from dogs and could relax into a more companionable stance.

The instinctive centre of *canine companioning*, or some dogs' seemingly unschooled ability to sit with a human 'side by side' can be seen in therapy modalities that employ dogs. Our family dog, Duffy, has this remarkable talent, seasoned with self-styled seduction: if a guest feels anxiety with dogs, Duffy remains determinedly composed and quietly *companions* the visitor, blinking benignly, but moving methodically closer, paw step by paw step. By the visit's end, Duffy's large furry body is inevitably draped across the smitten friend's lap – no words are necessary.

Unlike any matrix of *companioning* between humans – where detours or cycles of discord inevitably occur to threaten the relationship's survival, we may feel frustrated with a dog's undesirable behaviour, but we can rest upon our knowledge of their positive regard. Until the animal dies!

Todd

Unlike Eric, Todd is sophisticated and well-educated, with extensive experience in psychoanalysis. Like Eric, Todd requires my 'implicit relational knowing' (Stern et al., 1998, p. 907) because he 'harbour[s] self-states that contain earlier, undeveloped, unspeakable and non-related parts...that can find no expression in language' (ibid, p. 3). He too camouflages unformed states of illusion and merger intrinsic to his imagined narcissistic relationship with his dog.

Five years ago, when Todd was thirty-seven, his German Pointer, Siggy, dies, and I receive a referral from his now-retired analyst. Todd describes a major depression that lingers following Siggy's loss. As Todd's 'best friend' Siggy had accompanied Todd to his canine-friendly office, run with him every day along the river, and in summer, retrieved the sticks Todd threw into the Atlantic Ocean's choppy waters. 'Siggy,' he brags wistfully, 'swam like Michael Phelps.'

A hip looking, creative director at an advertising firm in Manhattan, Todd is always well dressed, immaculately groomed, with hair that is prematurely greyed at the temples, giving him a substantial presence that defies his years. He has an outsized, throaty laugh, which I find appealing. Now living alone, Todd wanders in and out of relationships with amiable women who mean little to him other than as a brief sexual encounter or as a date for a work event. He complains of fatigue and worries that his peers have all married, while he remains alone – without Siggy. His father's serious cardiovascular condition causes Todd inordinate stress, and he worries about his mother's becoming emotionally reliant on him in the future.

Todd's former analyst characterizes him as 'deeply intelligent but narcissistic'. The remark makes me initially feel protective of Todd, although he can be unquestionably grandiose. He earned his narcissistic stripes within a consistently unresponsive family system. His father is at times verbally vicious, and his mother is continually disengaged and passive. His privileged background gains him admission to a prestigious arts programme at an Ivy League college, where he finds psychic refuge for both his intellectual curiosity and athleticism, but the women he meets are conventional and incurious like his mother. Upon returning to New York City, he begins psychoanalysis and now sits slumped in my office.

'Siggy required enormous exercise, as do I. He was a real jock, what my father praised as a "manly" dog, a rare acknowledgment,' Todd stifles a sob. 'He slept on my bed and always knew whenever I had a gruelling day at work. He'd just dose if I was watching TV, his head in my lap.' Todd's tearful recounting seemed to bring both of them alive. Now, he tells me, he frequents a nearby dog run – 'looking like a paedophile at a playground'.

Todd confidently relied on Siggy's *canine companioning* with its all-purpose twinship relevance, seamlessly fitting into Todd's life. Due to Todd's insecure attachment style, he found it difficult to build and sustain ties with romantic companions, and he was initially suspicious of me. Todd's mother stifles any show of affection for him, seemingly anxious about his father's dissatisfaction with her, and his early warning to her – within Todd's earshot – that 'women like you inadvertently create homosexual sons'. 'At least she had the good sense to hire a caring nanny', Todd remarks wistfully. His selfobject experiences throughout his life – with teachers, colleagues, and his analyst – were ways in which Todd constructed emotional scaffolding outside of his family, and he remains remote from his formal, unwelcoming parents although they live in the same city.

I worry that I am now a designated nanny or perhaps a new Siggy, which is more to my liking. I need to '*companion*' Todd, listening with dogged empathy as he tells me innumerable 'Siggy stories' of unparalleled feats. Siggy was named for Dr. Freud, whom Todd describes as a kind of 'uber-nanny'. Beyond unwavering attention, can I be companionable enough to form a bridge to some future human partnership?

Todd is seriously dating Janna before Siggy's death, but he feels in no shape to discuss marriage with her. We talk about Janna's ability to provide him with Siggy's seemingly incalculable functions, and I think to myself that they are well-matched after Todd introduces us at one of his sessions. The couple marries and decides to have children right away, largely because Janna is in her late thirties, and Todd is fixed upon a fantasy of his own re-parenting.

Fast forward: Todd is now forty-two and looks very worried. Marriage to Janna has proven 'astonishing,' and, 'more than he could hope for'. She is a doctor who is taking time off to care for their daughter, Amy, aged two. The couple is adopting two Pointer littermates, to 'round out' their current family system, and Todd insists that he feels happy and able to successfully 'love and work'. But instead of experiencing a lift in his spirits at the thought of finally having everything he had missed as a child, he begins to have disturbing dreams in which Siggy demeans Janna, in words and behaviours – like barking incessantly at her so that Todd awakens. Janna, herself in therapy, feels perplexed by Todd's mood change, and urges him to, 'go talk to Ginny. I haven't seen you like this since Siggy died. You're not sleeping, you're barely eating and you've lost that client who you felt was solid. I'm worried'. Todd now heads up a small, multinational ad agency. 'Sounds impressive, right' he had grinned stoically at me. I roll my eyes and laugh gently, but wonder with questioning eyes about what anxieties have raised Siggy from the dead?

Todd and Janna both want a dog. She had had dogs in her Midwest childhood and wants another, 'I think more than she wants another kid', Todd teases, when he tells me she is again pregnant; this time with a boy about whom he is thrilled as much as he enjoys Amy. 'These dreams make no sense; how can I think that Siggy is displeased with Janna? Siggy had liked her, wagging his tail at her emphatically.' But Todd knows that these dreams are his own psychological constructions, and his underlying worries or defences belie his distrust that life can continue purposefully and contentedly with a human partner.

After Todd's father has a serious heart attack, a pacemaker is inserted but keeps malfunctioning, causing his mother to 'fall apart'. She tells Todd that she had always acquiesced to his dad because 'I didn't think I could live without him – I guess I really can't. But please let me make up for what I didn't do for you as a child'. Todd blows up, warning his mother that she cannot manipulate her way into his good graces. 'I spent all of this time thinking that it was all him', he tells me. 'She's a manipulating bitch! No wonder Father came home late every night', sounding un-Todd-like. 'Yeah, that was harsh', he admits. 'Dad probably wanted to marry a pretty girl from a prosperous family, and she was that'. We delve into Todd's feelings around his anger, so long restrained and finally unleashed.

In a later session, I take a deep breath and check Todd's mood to see if he has calmed down enough to hear me. 'I'd like to mention something that I've been wondering about and if it makes sense to you. I don't believe that Siggy could dislike Janna any more than you do. And I think your expectation that the puppies will 'round out your family' may be worrisome, causing you to search for reasons to project your unconscious fears about them onto your wife. What if the puppies disappoint you or the children? What if they're unable to be wonderful companions like Siggy had been? What will happen if one dies? Will you experience the complex mourning that you felt after Siggy died? You know intellectually that it will be an entirely different experience. Janna seems to provide you the closeness and comradeship like Siggy's, plus a healthy dose of sex', I smile. 'The feeling of Siggy is always with you Todd – he's not replaceable. Does that make any sense?' He nods. When we reconvene, Todd simply smiles at me and replies, 'You were right on'. The puppies arrive and are raucously silly, bringing the expanding family much laughter. The couple's son, Evan, is born, and Todd and Janna dream of a third child and perhaps a move to the country.

Todd's Achilles heel is his mistrust of becoming dependant on people, having early on disbelieved his parents' caring about him. Only Siggy, a non-human, could be emotionally unswerving and companionable. This case illustrates an often-missed element in classical analyses: that of 'being with' in a distinctive empathic and intersubjective manner as opposed to concentration on symbolically restructuring preconscious experience. It highlights the intensely affective requirement in a relationally shared space or third (Benjamin, 2004). In this treatment, we co-create access to early deficits, work through inevitable enactments in the therapy and among family members, but not necessarily in that order. '*Companioning*' stays in the moment to moment evolution of Grossmark's 'flow of enactive engagement', a resoluteness that can be critical in complicated mourning like Todd's.

Anthropomorphism

Humans have participated in anthropomorphic mythologizing since ancient times – when dogs were sometimes sacred ancestors or totems. The early Greeks' three-headed dog, Cerebus, guarded the underworld's doorway and a dog is the only being to recognize Odysseus when he returns from his legendary travels. Nearly as myth-like, Snoopy, the enigmatic beagle in the Peanuts' comic family, exhibits his artist's anthropomorphising, and innumerable other animals parade through each *New Yorker* issue.

Anthropomorphism is defined as the attribution of human qualities to non-humans and anthropopathism is the granting of human feelings to non-humans: each is ubiquitous. This behaviour literally animates conventional lives and offers metaphoric benefits to us. In today's perplexing world, it is common to name your car, or to curse your malfunctioning computer for failing to obey your commands. Anthropomorphising stokes creativity and denial concurrently, so that although we consciously understand that anthropomorphising our dogs is self-indulgent and irrational, our wanting to know and not know simultaneously is not uncommon. Like a child listening to a fairy tale, we know and don't know if the witch will eat the children.

Ferenczi (1956) claims that 'the child passes through the animistic period...in which every object appears to him to be endowed with life' (p. 193). Without this capability, a child, say (Ulman and Paul, 2006, p. 338) can 'suffer a serious developmental arrest'. Ideally, their 'capacity for mastery' (ibid, p. 339) over non-human objects can later be reinvested in the adult world, morphing into the ability to play, create and appreciate cultural phenomena. But it differs from transitional experiencing however because childlike animism can continue 'to endow spontaneity...far beyond infancy' (Akhtar, 2003, p. 4). The 'capacity for mastery' Grolnick, Barkin, & Muensterberger, (in Akhtar, ibid, p. 5) say, is decathected and over time lies in 'limbo', instead of being forgotten like a transitional object.

Infantile animism may be re-established with an autonomous animal for which one also cares –a pet. Freud (1946, 1955) believes that as a child matures, he begins to accept *anthropocentrism,* the philosophical view arguing that people are the principal animals on Earth and our status requires us to act as guardians for the so-called lesser species, which is of course a Biblical precept.

Animals who speak in children's stories provide 'safe spaces' (Fustich, 2016, p. 13) for young minds because children perceive them as equals says Freud (1946, 1957), although they are designated purveyors of important adult-initiated, ethical principles and complex ideas. Approximately half (to my count) of Caldecott Medals, the children's literary prize, include dogs or cats as significant characters.

Most adults, particularly those having a close relationship with a relational creature, readily anthropomorphise to varying degrees – simply because it is pleasurable. For our patients, ascribing disproportionate anthropomorphic qualities to their relational creatures can, however, become a clinical facet of the treatment. Freeman (2005) talks of 'pets as transference objects, [that] can symbolically represent characteristics of idealised or demonised self or object representations …projections of dissociated aspects of one's self… aggressive impulses …assertive impulses and wishes…or sexual impulses… not-me scapegoats…surrogate victims, or trickster figures' (ibid, p. 34).

Mary

I treated Mary, a newly widowed young woman, who presented with passionate feelings about her two small Cocker Spaniels. She feels socially insufficient in the United States having lived in Beirut for six years after marrying a Lebanese man whom she met at university in England. Soon after her husband's sudden death, Mary fled Lebanon. Her administrative job at the American Embassy had ended, and currently, she has no desire to seek employment.

Mary's mischievously endearing pups accompany her to our sessions and vie for our attention creating chaos in their wake. They take turns on and off and under the couch while nipping at one another and leaving a trail of fur behind them. Although I am sometimes annoyed with the dogs' behaviour, Mary's insistence tells me how important it is for her to show me her pride in them and her good 'mothering'. Mary is often consumed by her childless situation. It helps when acquaintances chat with Mary as she sits with the dogs at outdoor cafes and during their daily walks in Central Park, helping her to feel less alone. They are her *twinship* and *alterego selfobjects*.

Mary's unceasing conversation with her dogs, called Lucy and Desi, leaves me in reverie about a satirical canine-inspired reality show – for this is indeed Mary's reality. The pups are costumed in an extensive array of fashionable coats, booties or Halloween costumes. Pink bows are fastened to Lucy's ear so that she is always known as the little girl dog.

When Desi becomes ill and must remain at the veterinarian's, Lucy, much like Mary, is noticeably upset when they arrive one afternoon for a 'crisis' session. Sitting uncharacteristically upright and still on Mary's lap, Lucy captures my eye contact and barks, no 'talks', with great distress, seeming to recount her worries about her brother. Her 'language' mimics Mary's cadence, rhythm and urgency, woof, woofing her grave concerns as Mary and

I sit dumfounded and immobilized in amazement. Our projections perhaps, but the dog's 'speech', sounding so much akin to Mary's, even via canine vocal apparatus, is unmistakable. So, with a little forethought, Lucy and I have a session; I address Lucy but try to respectfully explore Mary's anxiety, while she sits like a ventriloquist armed with a small furry dummy. During our multi-subjective, folie à trios I allot Lucy more attention than I often give Mary. As the interpersonalist Edgar Levinson often asks (2018, personal communication), 'what's going on around here?'

When Desi returns home the following day, the dogs re-establish bedlam in my office – as if nothing has changed, but Mary and I remain astonished, having co-witnessed something neither of us entirely understands. This scenario offers a breaking through of unidentified barriers in our work, formerly established by my eccentric boundaries and Mary's excessive anthropomorphising, and it opens up new dialogue sprinkled with laughter.

I tell my colleague Ellen about this experience after she adopts a new terrier named Zoë. She dismisses my story, saying congenially, 'Oh Zoë does that too. It's adorable', 'Sure Zoë does it', I think sarcastically. But then Ellen mails me a video of Zoë 'talking' to her cat when Zoë 'demands' attention; the cat responds by hissing and running off.

Is anthropomorphism de rigueur due to the state of our shared disquiet in the world? Perhaps, but it is also a blind spot in the analytic investigation. Stam & Kalmanovitch (1998) explain that the wide acceptance of experimental animal psychology during the advent of the last century altered animals' status – becoming abstractions and 'organisms of convenience' (p. 1135) calling E. L. Thorndike's introduction of measurable data replaced 'anthropomorphism, anecdotalism and introspection' (ibid). His application of 'scientific,' 'mechanistic' and 'progressive' (ibid) properties to laboratory animals moved his research with children into the 'laboratories' of mass educational settings, creating a hierarchical research ladder from an animal to a child to an adult. As lab animals became fundamental to twentieth-century modernism, Darwin's ideas slid into slumber, and anthropomorphism's subjective meanings are now seldom explored.

Unconditional love

The rap icon, Tupac Shakur's (1999) song 'Unconditional Love' speaks to the universal human longing for unconditional love:

> (What y'all want?)
> Unconditional Love (no doubt)
> Talking 'bout the stuff that don't wear off
> It don't fade
> It'll last for all these crazy days
> These crazy nights
> Whether you wrong or you right…

Shakur is correct; unconditional love is what we all want, but it cannot be scientifically authenticated. Those of us who are lucky enough to 'feel' its close proximity – whether from man or beast – are indeed fortunate.

Individuals like Mary often crave the unconditional love that her dog supplies. A twinship selfobject relationship with a relational creature jump-starts the potential for renewed emotional development (Tolpin, 1997), or a dog can act as a placeholder, as Siggy actively does for Todd and Leonardo does as a fetish for Evie. When severe relational malattunement or abuse is the norm in childhood, or when grief blindfolds the possibility of risking human relationships as it does for Mary, unconditional love can feel indispensable. However, its longing often indicates an inability to entertain and endure the limitations and disappointments inherent in all important relationships, human or canine, although during a period of complicated grief, it can maintain the psyche's equilibrium. If unconditional love is insisted upon, however, as it is with merger selfobject demands in therapy, it ensures one's belief in a singular, magical self-worth – as Eric hopes for as he rescues pit bulls.

Summary

While literary minds – from Thomas Mann and Anton Chekov to Jack London and John Steinbeck – have constructed numerous and important ways to illustrate the human-canine bond, our lack of available psychoanalytic language regarding these important attachments, I feel, increasingly interferes with our clinical discourse. I have recommended the use of *relational creatures* to refer to our canine companions and our communication with them as *a meeting of affects.* New means of explication are necessary if we are to understand these interspecies alliances.

And so I borrow Anthony Bass's (2015, p. 701) query to clinicians, which also serves to encapsulate the human beings' desire to comprehend their relationships with their dogs: Bass asks, 'Why [do] analysts and patients seem so regularly to have experiences of such deep, even uncanny points of connection, challenging ordinary assumptions about what we are capable of knowing and perceiving about each other?' Rephrasing his question, I ask: Why do humans seem to experience these same inscrutable and enigmatic states of being with their relational creatures? Can we please begin a discussion?

References

Akhtar, S. (2003) Things: Developmental, psychopathological, and technical aspects of inanimate objects. *Canadian Journal of Psychoanalysis*, 11(1), pp. 1–44.

Akhtar, S. and Brown, J. (2005) Animals in psychiatric symptomatology. In S. Akhtar and V. Volkan (Eds.), *Mental zoo: Animals in the human mind and its pathology* (pp. 3–38). Madison, CT: International Universities Press.

Akhtar, S. and Volkan, V. (2005) *Mental zoo: Animals in the human mind and its pathology* (pp. 3–38). Madison, CT: International Universities Press.

American Pet Products Association. (2019–2020) *APPA National Pet Owners Survey, Breakdown of pet ownership in the U.S.* viewed 3 June 2019. https://www.american petproducts.org/press_industrytrends.asp.

Aron, L. (1996) *A meeting of minds.* Mahwah, NJ: Analytic Press.

Atsma, A. J. (2000–2019) The Kynokephaloi (Cynocephali) in Greek mythology. *Theoi Project, Classical Texts Library.* viewed 21 May 2018. https://www.theoi. com/Phylos/Kunokephaloi.html.

Baker, R. (1984) Some considerations arising from the treatment of a patient with necrophilic fantasies in late adolescence and young adulthood. *International Journal of Psycho-Analysis*, 65, pp. 283–294.

Bass, A. (1991) Fetishism, reality, and "The snow man." *American Imago*, 48(3), pp. 295–328.

Bass, A. (2015) It takes one to know one; or whose unconscious is it anyway? *Psycho-analytic Dialogues*, 11(5), pp. 683–702.

Beebe, J. (1997) Attitudes toward the unconscious. *Journal of Analytic Psychology*, 42(1), pp. 3–20.

Benjamin, J. (2004) Beyond doer and done to. *Psychoanalytic Quarterly*, 73(1), pp. 5–46.

Berns, G., Brooks, A. M. and Spivak, M. (2012) Functional MRI in awake, unre-strained dogs. *PLoS One*, 7(5). viewed 9 September 2018. https://journals.plos. org/plosone/article?id=10.1371/journal.pone.0038027.

Botiqué, L. R., Song, S. and Scheu, A. (2017) Ancient European dog genomes reveal continuity since early Neolithic. *Nature Communications*, 8, 16082. viewed 17 May 2019. https://www.ncbi.nlm.nih.gov/pubmed/28719574.

Brill, A. A. (1943) The universality of s symbols. *Psychoanalytic Review*, 30(1), pp. 1–18.

Brothers. D. (1993) The search for the hidden self: A fresh look at alterego transfer-ences. *Progress in Self Psychology*, 9, pp. 191–207.

Bulletin of the Anna Freud Centre. (1983) Personal Tributes (to Anna Freud). *Bulle-tin of the Anna Freud Centre*, 6(1), pp. 51–105.

Curnutt, K. (1999) Inside and outside: Gertrude Stein on identity, celebrity, and authenticity. *Journal of Modern Literature*, 23(2), pp. 291–308.

Darwin, C. (1998) *The expression of the emotions in man and animals.* London: Oxford Press.

Detrick, D. W. (1986) Alterego phenomena and the alterego transferences: Some further considerations. *Progress in Self Psychology*, 2, pp. 299–304.

Ferenczi, S. (1956) Stages in the development of the sense of reality. In C. Newton (Trans.) *Sex in psychoanalysis & the development of psychoanalysis* (pp. 181–202). New York: Dover.

Fletcher, J. (2007) Seduction and the vicissitudes of translation: The work of Jean Laplanche. *Psychoanalytic Quarterly*, 76(4), pp. 1241–1291.

Freeman D. M. A. (2005) Cross-cultural perspectives on the bond between man and animals. In S. Akhtar and V. Volkan (Eds.), *Cultural zoo: Animals in the human mind and its sublimations* (pp. 3–39). Madison, CT: International Universities Press.

Freud, A. (1995). Anna Freud in her own words: Devised by Ruth Rosen to cel-ebrate the centenary of Anna Freud. *Bulletin of the Anna Freud Centre*, 18(4), pp. 293–308.

Freud, S. (1946) *Totem and taboo*. New York: Vintage Books.

Freud, S. (1957) A difficulty in the path of psycho-analysis. *SE XVII*, pp. 135–144.

Freud, S. (1961). Fetishism. *SE XXI*, pp. 147–158.

Freud, S. (1962) *Three essays on the theory of sexuality*. In J. Strachey (Trans.). New York: Basic Books.

Fustich, K. (2016) The child-animal bond and the ethical functions of anthropomorphic children's literature. *Animal Studies*, Final research paper New York University.

Gay, P. (1988) *Freud: A life for our time*. New York: Doubleday.

Goldberg, J. R. and Mitchell, S. A. (2000) *Object relations in psychoanalytic theory*. Cambridge, MA: Harvard University Press.

Greenacre, P. (1955) Further considerations regarding fetishism. *Psychoanalytic Study of the Child*, 10, pp. 187–194.

Greenacre, P. (1969) The fetish and the transitional object. *Psychoanalytic Study of the Child*, 24, pp. 144–164.

Grossmark, R. (2018) *The unobtrusive relational analyst*. London: Routledge.

Heiman, M. (1956) The relationship between man and dog. *Psychoanalytic Quarterly*, 25, pp. 568–585.

Jones, E. (1957) *Sigmund Freud life and work 3: The last phase, 1919–1939* (pp. 1–521). London: Hogarth Press.

Jung, A. (2011) The grandfather. *Journal of Analytic Psychology*, 56(5), pp. 653–667.

Jung, C. G. (1989) *Memories, dreams and reflections*. In R. Winston and C. Winston (Trans.) and A. Jaffe (Ed.). New York: Vintage Press.

Kohut, H. (1971) *The analysis of the self*. Madison, CT: International Universities Press.

Kohut, H. (1977) *The restoration of the self*. New York: International Universities Press.

Kohut, H. (1984) *How does analysis cure?* In A. Goldberg and P. Stepansky (Eds.). Chicago, IL: University of Chicago Press.

Marcus, P. (2007) "I'm Just Wild about Harry!" A psychoanalyst reflects on his relationship with his dog. *Psychoanalytic Review*, 94(4), pp. 639–656.

Rawlings, M. K. (1966) *The yearling*. New York: Charles Scribner's Sons.

Richards, A. K. (1993) Perverse transference and psychoanalytic technique: An introduction to the work of Horacio Etchegoyen. *Journal of Clinical Psychoanalysis*, 2(4), pp. 463–480.

Schore, A. (2003) *Affect regulation and the repair of the self*. New York: Norton.

Searles, H. F. (1960) *The non-human environment in normal development and schizophrenia*. New York: International Universities Press.

Shakur, T. (1999) *Unconditional love*. Johnny "J" (Producer). Los Angeles, CA: Amaru, Death Row, Interscope Records.

Stam, H. J. and Kalmanovitch, T. (1998) E. L. Thorndike and the origins of animal psychology: On the nature of the animal in psychology. *American Psychologist*, 53(10), pp. 1135–1144.

Stern, D. N., Sander, L. W., Nahum, J. P., Harrison, A. M., Lyons-Ruth, K., Morgan, A. C., Bruschweilerstern, N. and Tronick, E. Z. (1998) Non-interpretive mechanisms in psychoanalytic therapy: The 'something more' than interpretation. *International Journal of Psycho-Analysis*, 79, pp. 903–921.

Stolorow, R. D. and Brandchaft, B. (1987). Developmental failure and psychic conflict. *Psychoanalytic Psychology*, 4(3), pp. 241–253.

Strozier, C. B. (2001) *Heinz Kohut: The making of a psychoanalyst.* New York: Farrar, Straus & Giroux.

Teasdale, D. S. (Ed.) (2010) *Dog Stories.* New York: Knoph.

Tolpin, M. (1971) On the beginnings of a cohesive self: An application of the concept of transmuting internalization to the study of the transitional object and signal anxiety. *The Psychoanalytic Study of the Child*, 26, pp. 316–352.

Tolpin, M. (1997) Compensatory structures: Paths to the restoration of the self. In A. Goldberg (Ed.), *Progress in self psychology* (Vol. 13, pp. 3–19). Hillsdale, NJ: Analytic Press.

Tolpin, M. (2007) The divided self: Shifting an intrapsychic balance the forward edge of a kinship transference: To bleed like everyone else. *Psychoanalytic Inquiry*, 27(1), pp. 50–65.

Ulman, R. B. and Paul, H. (2006) *The Self Psychology of addiction and its treatment: Narcissus in Wonderland.* New York: Routledge.

Winnicott. D. W. (1971) *Playing and reality.* London: Tavistock Publications.

Wolf, E. S. (1988) *Treating the self: Elements of clinical Self Psychology.* New York: Guilford Press.

Woolf, V. (1933) *Flush.* New York: Harcourt Brace.

Worboys, M., Strange, J. and Pemberton, N. (2018) *The invention of the modern dog: Breed and blood in Victorian England.* Baltimore, MD: Johns Hopkins University Press.

Young-Bruehl, E. (1988) *Anna Freud: A biography.* New York: WW Norton.

4 A dog in the room

Interspecies intersubjectivity in relational psychotherapy

Sean Meggeson

From Freud to the present day, therapists have had a tendency (and maybe a need) to either sentimentalise dogs and anthropomorphise their part in the therapeutic process or assign them the role of objects of identification, projection and displacement (Ponder, 2019). Both perspectives are limiting and unfair to dogs, making it seem like they are some kind of therapy toy: at best on the periphery of psychotherapeutic action, dogs are denied a sense of self and thereby excluded from the intersubjective field. Even though the past fifty years of Animal-Assisted Therapy has afforded a more agentive role of animals in the therapeutic process as authentic objects of attachment, and even as sole therapists (Levinson, 1984), I believe that more thinking, listening and development is needed on this topic and that relational therapists who include dogs in their practice can start thinking more radically about dogs in the room as participants in the intersubjective field.

The need for a 'dog turn' is especially relevant within the field of relational theory where the *Zeitgeist* of the nonverbal, as interpersonal theorist D.B. Stern puts it, has made it 'a little quaint to characterise psychoanalysis as the talking cure' (Stern, 2019, p. 68). For at least the last forty years, cognitive ethnologists, psychologists, philosophers and sociologists have done extensive research and analysis of inter-species intersubjectivity, concluding that a form of interspecies intersubjectivity *is* possible (Aaltola, 2013; Bekoff, 2003, 2006; Irvine, 2004, 2007; Jerolmack, 2009; Jürgens, 2017; Rowlands, 2019; Shapiro, 1990, 2003; Zlatev et al., 2008). This chapter will relate relational/intersubjective theory and clinical practice to some of the research on inter-species intersubjectivity, emphasising the importance of 'kinaesthetic empathy' (Shapiro, 1990, 2003) and the nonverbal. I will discuss how some unformulated (Stern, 2019) clinical moments in the client-canine-therapist triad become affected by the awareness of difficult shadow states of primal being. Finally, I will present a clinical example with my canine co-therapist, Tao-Tao ('Tao' for short; pronounced 'taow').

First, a few words on my co-therapist. Tao is an 11-kilogram Swedish Vallhund, a rare pure-bred herding dog that supposedly reaches back to the times of the Vikings. She has smiley lips, short legs and looks like a Corgi mated with a Husky. Tao is friendly and extremely calm, and while she can definitely bark if she wants to, she never does so while working in the consulting room. She has her own 'canine therapy' business card, but she is not a trained therapy dog. In sessions, her subjectivity is ever-present, encouraging clients' subjectivity to emerge. For example, when paying for a session, one client tried to tuck the cheque under Tao's collar, saying, 'Here, take this to the Master.' Another client broke some dog treats into little bits, laid them out like a buffet for a drooling Tao and said, 'Time for my interspecies love session'. Other clients have said things like: 'Well, at least Tao-Tao was a good listener today', 'Where's my little baby?!', 'Tao-Tao and I are having a staring contest—she's very aggressive', 'Oh, to be like Tao—so relaxed and care-free', 'I hope she doesn't vomit on the carpet again', 'She's so thin! Are you feeding her enough, Sean?' And on and on...While every verbal statement by a client might be worth analysing, interpretation that seeks understanding, of course, is not enough (Levinson, 1972).

Tao has taught me much about the value of being a non-invasive, kinaesthetically embodied dweller of nonverbal integrative therapeutic spaces. This kind of dwelling involves what psychologist and co-founder of the Animals and Society Institute, Kenneth Shapiro outlines as canine-defined bodily experiences made up of 'paths to be traversed, of territory staked out, of felt relations—all known implicitly and bodily' (Shapiro, 2003, p. 90). In other words, a canine therapist asks us to follow their example and de-emphasize verbal dyadic interchange, and to focus on what's happening in the body, between bodies. This is the canine-human intersubjective *modus operandi*. In the nonverbal territory of body-with-body, Tao offers moments of subtle affect, embodied messages, shifts, poses, pokes, licks and looks. For example, as a client settles into the session, Tao will usually sense where she needs to be spatially. After standing by me for a moment or two, Tao may move toward the client, have a quick sniff or lick at their ankle, and then sit by their feet. Tao will glance at the client, then at me and eventually she will settle herself—and wait. A client usually does not comment at length on Tao's presence, but sometimes will glance at Tao and say something like, 'Look— she's right here'. Somehow Tao knows where her place should be in the room, and consequently the best place to be in the therapeutic process: near or far; tactful or present; still or moving; waiting or ready. She can anticipate these positions by her use of implicit relational knowing, a knowing embedded in bodily experience.

When this process takes place and I'm attuned to it, I feel unusually grounded in the room in a strange, still and silent way that feels peaceful, but at the same time filled with readiness. Something akin to the spiritual meaning of the Taoist concept of *Wu Wei* that holds that action comes from inaction. In this place, I feel integrated and receptive to the client. The entire process—as it involves an intersubjective triad of therapist, dog and client—serves not as an analogy to relational psychotherapeutic process—it *is* the process.

Even though he never mentions dogs, D.B. Stern (2019) has much to say about unformulated/formulated nonverbal client material within the context of interpersonal/relational theory that can apply to working intersubjectively with a dog in the room. For Stern, the unformulated becomes formulated via language, and within the context of phenomenology, the human subject becomes realised through language and verbal dialogic processing as a meaning-making endeavour between people (Gadamer, 2013; Merleau-Ponty, 2013). This formulation would seem to exclude interspecies intersubjectivity—and in the verbal realm, it does. Yet, in *The Infinity of the Unsaid*, Stern admits that by focusing on the verbal as the primary element in the clinical field, the therapist misses much that is emergent and unbidden. In earlier work, Stern (1983, cited in 2019, p. 7) states, '[t]he unformulated must organize itself first. It must begin to coalesce...It must send up tendrils, or feelings of tendency'. A dog's tendrils are her very presence. A client looks at Tao in a moment of painful isolation and says with some relief, '*She* knows how I'm feeling'. And as a result, the client actually *feels* a connection with Tao by virtue of the dog's nonverbal presence—a feeling of tendency, kinship and connection based on the dog's present availability. Expert on animal emotions, Marc Bekoff, comments on the nature of the nonverbal intersubjective moment that exists between humans and all animals: 'As I watch an animal, I'm not reaching for the closest word to describe the behaviour I see; I'm feeling the emotion directly, without words or even a full, conscious understanding of the animal's actions' (Bekoff, 2007, p. 128). The power of this connection can be seen in the numerous clients who relate how their painful childhoods were made bearable by such human-to-animal moments.

The nonverbal process relates to the concept of procedural knowing (especially as it is described by Stern) within the context of nonverbal, affective therapeutic action. Stern (2019) explains, '[p]rocedural knowing has no symbolic form in the mind, and is defined by what it does...Examples with psychoanalytic relevance include various affective, prosodic, visual and auditory sensory-perceptual, kinaesthetic, motor, and social-interactive phenomena—the stuff of somatic experience...' (p. 22). Also, as Stern says, it is working within the realm of the procedurally-organized that change happens. A dog in the room offers clients nonverbal and connected ways to re-attune to the procedural and hence, to hidden, split-off affects.

'Feelings of tendency' is an apt way to describe the implicit knowledge and feelings, the nonverbal presence that dogs offer humans who feel isolated in their quest for the relational meeting. In the psychotherapeutic process, these nonverbal events of feelings of tendency between dog and client add to the therapeutic action in relational work. Stern (ibid) states, 'I believe that nonverbal events are, in a certain sense, primary in the creation of therapeutic action' (p. 16). They *are* primary, and they touch upon something elemental, primitive, and, I would argue, shadow-like.

The nonverbal asks us to consider our mammalian animal-body without the social overlay of verbal language. In this difficult awareness resides primal shadow parts of nonverbal human subjectivity. While the nonverbal can be an integrative space of containment and holding, it can also be a mysterious, complex and sometimes unstable state of being that compels all living things and unites us with the dog. In 1936, Dutch Psychologist and phenomenologist F.J.J. Buytendijk wrote in *The Mind of a Dog*, '[t]he most profound secret of life lies in the dual aspect of all its relations. [...] The entire animal world [including humans] calls for and responds to the desire for appeasement, peace, and deliverance from its loneliness' (Buytendijk, 1936, pp. 19–21). The dog howls from loneliness; the human dog tends to forget the felt meaning of this nonverbal articulation, a procedural plea toward a meeting that holds the hope of deliverance. Buytendijk (ibid, pp. 14–15) adds,

> Is not the joy of meeting ever like a *Wiedersehen*, just as if each had known the other in a former life? It is like this, too, with man (sic) and dog. Neither has a guaranteed place in Nature, both are exiles. No two animals in the inmost recesses of their nature seek each other so earnestly and attach themselves to each other as do these.

Both human and dog need each other no less than human needs human, the genesis and *telos* of all therapeutic action.

As informed relational psychotherapists, it is both Tao's and my task to meet a client's needs for connection, even in the shadow realms of the nonverbal. This may mean departing from the traditional phenomenological task of assisting the unformulated toward formulation. Rather, it requires staying in the primal, felt a moment of howling and leaving the unformulated within the nonverbal realm of felt knowledge. In this sense, *talk* therapy with a dog in the room becomes at times defunct in the presence of procedural knowledge and its grounding action for all animals. And perhaps in certain, crucial events of body-with-body interchanges, the talking of talk therapy *should* remain in abeyance, privileging nonverbal interspecies intersubjectivity— no language, symbols, signs, or emergent properties within the linguistic matrix; rather, an inter-species intimation of unified being.

Clinical example

Jenny (a pseudonym) is a thirty-year-old woman who up until the time of this clinical example had been in treatment with me for about a year and a half. As a result of developmental deprivations and cumulative relational trauma, Jenny struggles with self and mutual regulation. She does not trust her own body and does not trust others'. In early treatment, Jenny would have panic attacks and would self-harm. These attacks were brought on by on-going relational injuries and deprivations, accumulated work stress, as well as catastrophic thinking and death anxiety. While we had a good working relationship, Jenny's self-structure was such that any regulating connection I offered (verbal and nonverbal) was transformed into confirmation of her shame, triggering an attack on self and our relationship. She rapidly unravelled in early treatment and spent a month in a government psychiatric hospital where she tried to commit suicide. Upon release, we continued sessions and she improved over the months.

Her relationship with Tao has been implicitly ambivalent. Jenny likes Tao, but when Tao becomes bothersome to her (especially with Tao's insistent licking of ankles), Jenny pushes Tao away rather callously. Tao has taken the hint and keeps a respectful distance. She generally refrains from licking Jenny in favour of offering distant kinaesthetic empathy, usually finding a spot equidistant from Jenny and me, but facing Jenny.

During a session in which we were discussing a difficult aspect of her hospitalisation, Jenny began having a panic attack as she sat on the couch. Her eyes filled with terror, her body constricted in on itself, and her voice became young. With her head bowed and shoulders hunched, Jenny squeaked out the words, 'Can you please sit with me on the couch?' I froze and tried to formulate a sentence that would somehow make Jenny feel okay, but also give me an excuse not to sit with her on the couch. I did not want to be close to her animal fear and while I did not articulate it consciously to myself at that moment, I was afraid of her fear. Yet, another part of me knew words would not be enough and I needed to sit next to her. Sit *with* her in her fear, loneliness and chaos.

I took a quick breath and readied myself to move to the couch. As I stood up from my chair, Tao stood too and glanced at me with readiness. And in the same action of moving toward Jenny, I scooped up Tao and carried her with me to the couch, placing her half on my lap and half on Jenny's. As the three of us settled into that shared space of panic and fear, I could feel Tao's body become relaxed. Feeling unused to such physical proximity to a client, I said nothing, and Jenny began to slowly pet Tao on her scruff. Tao became even more relaxed and it seemed to me, grew discernibly warmer in her under-belly. Tao then began to gently lick Jenny's hand as she petted her scruff. Jenny allowed Tao to keep licking. As I felt Tao's relaxed closeness, I began to say softly, 'It's okay, it's okay...' Both Jenny and I needed these 'words.' But they were less words than nonverbal sounds, a rhythmical demarcation of a safe space.

With Tao holding the intersubjective triad, I sensed that Jenny was arcing out of the panic attack. The three of us then sat in intimate silence for a spacious moment. I then intuitively looked at Jenny and asked, 'Good?'. She shyly looked at me and nodded, 'Yes.' When I stood up, Tao jumped off the couch, and when I returned to my chair, Tao sat by my feet. The only thing Jenny said about this event was in the next session: 'All I remember was your voice was gentle. And Tao really helped.'

Conclusion

Artist and ecological scholar, Uta Maria Jürgens has claimed, 'Intersubjectivity across species boundaries is the experiential stuff from which relationality is made' (Jürgens, 2019, p. 27). Accordingly, a dog in the room is not merely an object of projection, identification and displacement. A dog in the room participates in an interspecies intersubjective triad that is kinaesthetically empathic and nonverbal. Furthermore, a canine co-therapist urges relational psychotherapists to think more deeply about psychotherapeutic action as it relates to somatic groundedness, specifically within the context of nonverbal, unformulated material, which can include the awareness and mutual regulation of a difficult shadow state of being.

Finally, as mentioned, Tao always seems to find her place in the room and then reconsiders her place appropriately. In this, she communicates to me the value of reconsidering *my* position in the room and how changing places, especially in the presence of loneliness, fear and chaos, can facilitate growth and healing for both the client and me.

References

Aaltola, E. (2013) Empathy, intersubjectivity and animal philosophy. *Environmental Philosophy,* 10 (2), pp. 1–36.

Bekoff, M. (2003) Minding animals, minding earth: Science, nature, kinship, and heart. *Human Ecology Review,* 10 (1), pp. 56–76.

Bekoff, M. (2006) *Animal passions and beastly virtues: Reflections on redecorating nature.* Philadelphia, PA: Temple University Press.

Bekoff, M. (2007) *The emotional lives of animals: A leading scientist explores animal joy, sorrow, and empathy—and why they matter.* Novato, CA: New World Library.

Buytendijk, F.J.J. (1936) *The mind of a dog.* Translated by L.A. Clare. Boston, MA and New York: Houghton Mifflin.

Gadamer, H.G. (2013) *Truth and method.* London: Bloomsbury Academic.

Irvine, L. (2004) *If you tame me: Understanding our connection with animals.* Philadelphia, PA: Temple University Press.

Irvine, L. (2007) The question of animal selves: Implications for sociological knowledge and practice. *Qualitative Sociology Review,* 3 (1), pp. 5–22.

Jerolmack, C. (2009) Humans, animals, and play: Theorizing interaction when intersubjectivity is problematic. *Sociological Theory,* 27 (4), pp. 371–389.

Jürgens, U.M. (2017) How human-animal relations are realized: From respective realities to merging minds. *Ethics & the Environment,* 22 (2), pp. 25–57.

Levinson, B. (1984) Human/companion animal therapy. *Journal of Contemporary Psychotherapy,* 14 (2), pp. 131–144.

Levinson, E.A. (1972) *The fallacy of understanding: An inquiry into the changing structure of psychoanalysis.* New York, NY: Basic Books.

Merleau-Ponty, M. (2013) *Phenomenology of perception.* New York, NY: Routledge.

Ponder, J. (2019) Patients use of dogs as objects of identification, projection, and displacement. *Psychoanalytic Psychology,* 36 (1), pp. 29–35.

Rowlands, M. (2019) *Can animals be persons?* Oxford: Oxford University Press.

Shapiro, K.J. (1990) Understanding dogs through kinaesthetic empathy, social construction and history. *Anthrozoos*, 3 (3), pp. 184–195.

Shapiro, K.J. (2003) What it is to be a dog: A qualitative method for the study of animals other than humans. *The Humanistic Psychologist*, 31 (4), pp. 67–96.

Stern, D.B. (2019) *The infinity of the unsaid: Unformulated experience, language, and the nonverbal.* New York, NY: Routledge.

Zlatev, J., Racine, T.P., Sinha, C. and Itkonen, E. (2008) Intersubjectivity: What makes us human? In J. Zlatev, T.P. Racine, C. Sinha and E. Itkonen, E. (Eds.), *The shared mind: Perspectives of intersubjectivity.* Amsterdam: Benjamins, pp. 1–14.

5   Someone to run with

Towards a relational neuroscientific approach to dog-assisted child psychotherapy

Dor Roitman

Grossman's beautiful novel 'Someone to run with' (2004) begins with these words:

> A dog runs through the streets; a boy runs after it. A long rope connects the two and gets tangled in the legs of the passersby, who grumble and gripe, and the boy mutters "Sorry, sorry" again and again. In between mumbled sorries he yells "Stop! Halt!" – and to his shame a "Whoa-ha!" escapes from his lips. And the dog keeps running (p. 3).

And somewhat later:

> Dinka walked beside him, her head bowed, her tail drooping; walking like that on the side of the road, they looked like two mourners. The rope dragged on the ground between them. Assaf opened his hand and let it fall to the ground, but Dinka stopped, as if she were amazed and scared by his action, from the hinted intention of it. Assaf immediately bent down and picked it up (p. 101).

In these two quotes, Grossman vividly encapsulates the deep emotional bond that a person and a dog can share, the multiple levels of implicit communication that flow both ways and the way they can regulate each other's emotional states. It is also a beautiful example of emotional contagion and of projective identification between human and non-human animals.

Animal Assisted Psychotherapy (AAP) is concerned with the effects of the presence of animals in a setting, which is used for the psychotherapy of humans. It builds on the way people and animals perceive, respond and interact with each other, to enhance the therapeutic process. People, especially children, are often strongly attracted to, cognitively intrigued by and emotionally responsive to animals. They are inclined to attribute a personality, intentionality and an inner emotional life to living beings from all species. For reasons that will become clearer further down, we humans easily connect with domesticated mammals such as dogs, relating to them as attachment figures, social partners, friends, siblings, offspring and so on.

Dogs are social relational beings, able to connect with other social animals and to build relationships with them. As I will show later, they share with us humans quite a similar neuro-physiological operating system that codes the interpersonal world in homologous tools and signals and operates in like mental and behavioural patterns. They, too, tend to see us, under the right conditions, as partners in creating and maintaining relational bonds. Hence, the participation of dogs in the analytic space brings with it an expansion of the possibilities for interactions and relationships for both the patient and therapist, within a more elaborate interpersonal matrix. Relational processes involving a third subject in the form of a dog in the analytic field occur as spontaneously as those involving the therapist and the patient.

A child therapist introducing a dog to the analytic space faces the challenge of dynamically administrating the therapeutic sessions accordingly while remaining engaged in the three-way interactions as they unfold, and at the same time being aware of and processing the multiple levels of communication and interaction that transpire, to the benefit of the therapeutic process. One question that constantly arises is about the ethical stance of the therapist and his/her responsibilities towards the dog. These (and other) issues and challenges require that we have a theoretical standpoint, to guide our clinical thinking and technique. Unfortunately, current theories on animal relationality and on dynamic psychotherapy in the presence of animals are scarce and insufficient. The first goal of this chapter is to propose some guidelines for such a theory. The second goal is to demonstrate how this theory can be applied in a therapeutic setting to guide the clinical assessment of and technical approach to the inclusion of a dog in the psychotherapy of children.

In the first part of this chapter, I will speak about what I think functions as a connecting tissue between all sentient beings, especially mammals. I refer here to specific mental and neurological mechanisms that I think belong to some aspects of the relational self. I will suggest that this level of functioning and communication is in the heart of dogs' and people's habits of seeing each other as similar and significant subjective others and to treat each other as legitimate partners for relational and interpersonal processes, as attachment figures and as transferential and transitional objects. This part will be dedicated to the establishment of the neuroscientific foundations for a clearer concept of the relational self in dogs. Based on this, in the second part of the chapter, using clinical material, I will demonstrate how the concept of relationality in dogs contributes to how we think about and work with what happens between a child patient and a dog in psychotherapy. Using the theoretical model that will be presented in the first part, some of the processes commonly explored in the relational literature and which are taking place in the human-animal matrix of the therapeutic session in which a dog is present will be discussed.

Discussing animal relationality and relational processes between humans and dogs necessitate, I think, a multi-disciplinary approach. A deep asymmetry is embedded in the dominating (some will say domineering) position that humans assume towards non-human animals. An exploration of the intrapsychic and subjective realm of dogs, in their relations with humans, might come across as projective and anthropomorphising and in any case be suspected to be over speculative. This is due to a disruption in the way we humans perceive the evolutionary continuity of which we are all a part, people and animals. Since I see this as a major problem that has impeded our theoretical advancement and creativity for many years, I decided to begin this chapter by reflecting on the human-animal split and the reasons for the lack of theory about animal relationality and intersubjective processes between humans and animals. In the present state of affairs, I think that in order to establish a sound and applicable relational approach to the effects of the presence of a dog in therapy, which takes into account such concepts as Self, Consciousness, Object Relations and Relationality, it is important that we base our premises on findings from various fields of knowledge. I found reinforcement in Schore's words, relating to what he sees as Bowlby's profoundly significant proposition, equally favoring an interdisciplinary approach to the study of developmental phenomena. Schore (2000) states that

> in such an approach the collaborative knowledge-bases of a spectrum of sciences would yield the most powerful models of both the nature of the fundamental ontogenetic processes that mediate the infant's first attachment to another [human] being, and the essential psychological mechanisms by which these processes indelibly influence the development of the organism at later points of the life-cycle (p. 24. My square brackets).

The reader may therefore find that this chapter speaks in more than one language. I hope that by connecting the dots I will be able, eventually, to draw a clear line around what I think could be a useful unified theoretical approach to Dog-Assisted Child Psychotherapy, and to offer therapists something to run with.

Part I: A relational neuroscientific theory of dog relationality

A disruption in the human-animal communal bond

Once upon a time, our ancestors, the Homo-Sapiens, emerged as a distinct species of the Hominid family, the great apes. This process involved the gradual development of capabilities such as bipedalism and language. At that time no scholars and philosophers were about to ponder upon the differences and similarities between this new evolving species and other kinds of animals. Many centuries later came the Hunter-Gatherer era, with its tribal culture. By that time, around 40,000 years ago, the extinction of the Neanderthals, the other subspecies of archaic humans in the genus Homo, was almost complete and Homo-Sapiens had largely established itself as the only human around. These early humans made marvellous discoveries, such as the taming of fire and wheat, developed elaborate ways of communicating abstract ideas through spoken and written language and achieved monumental feats through collaboration in big numbers. They realized that getting many people to cooperate was possible by convincing large populations to share in the belief in imagined stories about a world order, stories which functioned as social adhesives and motivational regulators (Harari, 2014). One question that these stories had to answer was – What makes us humans special, and what is the purpose of our being here? Many different answers were given to this question. A thread which was woven through all of them was the idea that there was something about humans that was essentially different from other non-human beings. Along the ages, this difference has expanded conceptually into a gulf, sustained by theological and later biological and psychological arguments. Freud, deeply influenced by the findings of Charles Darwin and the evolutionists, was puzzled by this change in man's attitude towards animals throughout life, as well as throughout our phylogenetic development. In 1917 he wrote:

> In the course of the development of civilization man acquired a dominating position over his fellow-creatures in the animal kingdom. Not content with this supremacy, however, he began to place a gulf between his nature and theirs. He denied the possession of reason to them, and to himself he attributed an immortal soul, and made claims to a divine descent which permitted him to break the bond of community between him and the animal kingdom... A child can see no difference between his own nature and that of animals... Not until he is grown up, does he become so far estranged from animals as to use their names in vilification of human beings.
>
> ...Man is not a being different from animals or superior to them; he himself is of animal descent, being more closely related to some species and more distantly to others. The acquisitions he has subsequently made have not succeeded in effacing the evidences, both in his physical structure and in his mental dispositions, of his parity with them (pp. 140–141).

Note his use of the expression 'the bond of community' (as translated by James Strachey), and the claim for parity in physical structure and mental dispositions. This passage can be read as suggesting the existence of a common matrix, incorporating both humans and non-humans, all connected through homologous physical and mental mechanisms. By now, a century after Freud's hypothesis, this idea has been robustly validated by research. I will refer later to some aspects of these findings.

Freud is also pointing here to what may be the main reason for still very persistent misconceptions about animals, which account for the fact that many of us are still reluctant to attribute feelings, personality and a subjective experience to animals. This is seen in the general avoidance in, among other places, the academic and clinical literature to address the animal's experience and point of view in its relationship with humans, or to analyse the human-animal interactions using psychoanalytic concepts and paradigms.

Animals are marginalized in the eyes and lives of humans (Berger, 1980). Berger says that pets have become mirrors for their owners, reflecting parts that need completion or recognition, taking the place of family members, representing trivial human traits and are raised to be 'creatures of their owner's way of life' (p. 14). In zoos, they are reduced to a spectacle, usually a disappointing one because in the zoo the animal is sedated, restricted, confined and stripped from its natural vigor and self-dependency. It rarely looks back at the visitors. Berger sensitively observes

> Therein lies the ultimate consequence of their marginalisation. That look between animal and man, which may have played a crucial role in the development of human society, and with which, in any case, all men had always lived until less than a century ago, has been extinguished (p. 28).

Myers (1998) also argues for the importance of re-centralizing the animals as they are in the actual lives of children, as a whole and compelling presence. In his criticism of psychoanalysis, Myers acknowledges that 'psychoanalytic theory assumes a biologically based commonality with animals, but this is normally expected to be transcended with development' (p. 38). And although there is an abundant reference to animals, he postulates, it is usually symbolic or projective representations belonging to immature parts of the human self, oedipal conflicts, antisocial urges, psychic stress or ill health. 'In therapy', he adds, 'they are but a means towards a mature social – that is to say, human – ego in a mono-species adult world' (p. 39). Myers believes, like I do, that in exploring the role of animals in human development, 'the key variable of interest, the child-animal relationship itself, needs to be the object of understanding' (p. 39).

So, as Myers puts it, 'Western culture may be exceptional in positing categorical human/nonhuman *contrasts*. Being human means *not* being an animal!' (Myers, 1998, p. 46. Italics in origin). It seems that under the cautious tendency not to anthropomorphise animals lies a deeply ingrained conviction that we humans are exclusive in possessing a subjective emotional life, next to an archaic fear of losing our long-cherished sense of superiority and uniqueness. Freud (1917) thought that after the cosmological blow, brought by the realization that the earth was not the stationary center of the universe, the evolutionary claim for a communal bond with our fellow creatures inhabiting this planet was the second severe blow to humanity's narcissistic self-love. Jaak Panksepp, a renowned researcher in (and founder of) Affective Neuroscience, reiterates, 'In my estimation, the argument against animal feelings comes ultimately from an unforgiving, anthropocentric form of solipsism combined with a pernicious form of neo-dualism' (Panksepp, 2001, p. 143).

Nowadays, though, mounting evidence from brain research and modern psychoanalytic theories is casting new light on human-animal relations. Following is a review of some selected findings and perspectives, which to my mind have consequential implications in this field. In presenting them in brief, I am proposing an evolutionistic approach which accepts that in evolution the new lies on top of the old, as epitomized in Darwin's notion of evolutional continuity, or in his dictum that the difference in the mental lives of animals are 'one of degree and not of kind' (Darwin, 1871, p. 105).[1] This also means that since the brain has retained evolutionary layering, 'lower' or more basic mental structures and functions will be found in a larger variety of species, or in other words, that 'from an evolutionary perspective... many of our fundamental abilities are remarkably similar to those of our brethren animals' (Panskepp, 2001, p. 144).

The relational self in dogs – exploring homologous mechanisms in animals

Subjective emotional experiences

In his exploration of the neurobiological substratum of emotions, Panskepp found evidence of genetically ingrained emotional systems, situated in deep subcortical areas of the brain, the arousal of which generates specific classes of emotional behavior and affective body-states (Panskepp, 2001, 2011, 2012). We can witness the operation of these mechanisms very easily in animals, on the behavioural level. Like when my dog Shula hears thunders on a stormy night and starts wailing and scratching the door in a desperate attempt to let herself in, or when my cat Itzik catches a glimpse of something moving in the grass and instantaneously crouches down flat with eyes and ears pointed forward. Affective neuroscience tells us that these behaviors are based on instinctual actions, or rather 'intentions in action', while at the same time the animal is experiencing a specific subjective feeling, an affective state or emotion, and a sense of valence (good or bad) which classifies the experience as potentially positive or negative in its effect on the survival of the organism (Panskepp, 2012).

Panskepp identified seven such primary-process emotional networks, correlated to specific neural circuits, which are: FEAR, RAGE, LUST, CARE, GRIEF, SEEKING and PLAY. The names of these distinct systems are capitalised for the purpose of differentiating them from the language of emotions that we regularly use (Panskepp, 2012). It helps to clear the distinction if we connect each emotion-action system to its prominent emotions, as in: RAGE – Anger, Hostility; FEAR – Anxiety, Fear, Dread; SEEKING – Enthusiasm, Expectancy; etc. We can now postulate that what was activated in Shula was the FEAR system, while in Itzik it was SEEKING.

Evidence also supports the claim that these mechanisms for affect are shared by all mammals and probably most vertebrates (Panskepp, 2001, 2012). What this means is that the capacity to feel affective emotions, accompanied by a clear sense of valence (good or bad), is an evolutionary forged ability shared by all mammals, including dogs. It can be easily explained how these mechanisms are necessary for survival.

Theories on the primary-self and core-consciousness

It seems then that this primordial level of functioning, these affective emotion-action mechanisms, are fundamental aspects of subjective experience. It follows that all mammals have subjective emotional experiences. What also seems to be implied from this is that we can speak about a neuro-biological self, a Primary SELF (Panskepp, 2012. Capitalised in origin.), or Proto-Self (Damasio, 1999), which is what binds, collects and weighs all these subjective affective-emotional experiences into an organismic coherence, or a continuous sense of an 'I', based on bodily sensations and representations. The biological self comes prior to the emergence of the narrative-self, or autobiographical-self in humans (and to some degree in other animals), which is the sense of 'who we are' based on memories, self-perceptions and projections into an anticipated future (Asma and Greif, 2012). The primordial biological self is centered in the coherent pre-verbal proprioceptive sense of the body and its survival needs and regulatory imperatives, which are the functions that Freud attributed to the Id and that Solms sees as the "fount of consciousness" (Solms, 2013, p. 5). What is this consciousness? As I see it, it is a continuous and automatic here-and-now evaluative assessment of sensory inputs from within and from without, regarding their relation to the individual organism and its survival. This is not a reflective-cognitive consciousness requiring more advanced cognitive capacities. It is closer to wakefulness than to awareness. Damasio (1999) equates 'core-consciousness' with 'feeling a feeling', in the sense that the organism has detected a change in its representation of its body state (the proto-self), and is able to produce 'representations of the proto-self as it is affected by interactions with a given environment' (p. 284).[2]

Stephen Asma and Thomas Greif (2012, pp. 30–31) tie it all together nicely:

> the self first emerges in the pre-cognitive ability of most organisms to operate from an egocentric point of view. Way below the level of propositional beliefs, animals must solve basic motor challenges (e.g. where am I in relation to that advancing sharp claw thing? Am I moving now, or is the environment moving? Am I eating my own arm?). For mammals this low-level ability is accompanied by the archetypical survival systems, shaped by natural selection over geological time. These are homological affective systems that Panskepp isolated in the brains and behaviors of his subjects: approach when SEEKING, escape from FEAR, attack in

RAGE mode, pursue nurturance in PANIC, seek mate in LUST mode, and so on. These affects and emotions are survival skills and comprise and pervade primary and secondary consciousness – they have to be 'owned' by the organism for them to work properly. This is why Panskepp and Damasio, both fans of Spinoza's monism, are in agreement about the reality of primary or core consciousness. Subjectivity resides first in the biological realm of action. It is not the disembodied Cartesian spectator.

We can therefore acknowledge the existence of a self in dogs, incorporating subjectively felt affective experiences and a core-consciousness able to detect changes in the embodied self, vis-à-vis external events, objects and stimuli.

Implicit communication and object-relating

Representations of changes in body state and of connections between affective experiences and environmental stimuli are the building blocks of procedural implicit knowledge. Implicit memory is where procedural knowledge is allegedly stored, and it is revealed when previous experiences facilitate performance on a task that does not require conscious or intentional recollection of those experiences (Graf and Schacter, 1985; Schacter, 1987). Implicit learning is fundamental in the learning processes of habituation and conditioning. In implicit learning, unconscious processes occur in which stored past experiences are reactivated and inform the way we interpret and respond to new experiences, creating over time (and repetition) new patterns of behavior. Conditioned emotions serve as an example of implicit memories. It has been found that the limbic system in the brain, and specifically the amygdala, plays a critical role in this type of learning/memory (Graf and Schacter, 1985). Fear conditioning in animals offers a reliable model of implicit learning, one where we already have a good understanding of the underlying neural circuitry.

Schore describes how implicit intersubjective affective transactions embedded in the attachment relationship with the mother influence the hard wiring of the emotion-processing areas in the infant's brain (Schore, 1994, 2005). Thus, implicit processing underlies the quick and automatic handling of nonverbal affective cues in infancy, by which attachment communication transpires. According to Schore and Schore, 'attachment experiences are thus imprinted in an internal working model that encodes strategies of affect regulation that act at implicit nonconscious levels' (2008, p. 12). Bowlby's original theory of attachment was based on ethological principles and observations (Bowlby, 1969). Attachment theory is widely accepted as referring to the infant-mother (and other attachment figures) relations in many animal species. A partial review of relevant literature can be found in Rajecki, Lamb and Obmascher (1978). Researches on dogs' attachment patterns towards humans found striking similarities with human attachment dynamics (Topal, Miklosi, Csanyi and Doka, 1998; Horn, Huber and Range, 2013).

The point I want to make here is that attachment behaviors and internal working models in dogs operate in similar ways as in humans. They are created through repeated implicit affective communication with the primary caretakers and are reactivated implicitly throughout life in social contexts. Earlier experiences thus influence the way dogs respond to humans, thereby reflecting their inner object-relating patterns. To reiterate, object-relating in dogs simply means that, like us, they are relating to significant others, including human others, according to their internalised representations of self and other and to their encoded strategies of affect regulation (working models) imprinted by early attachment experiences.

Regulation theory and the implicit-self-system

In considering neuroscientific findings with updated internal object relations theories, self-psychology, and contemporary relational theory, Schore and Schore (2008) offer a modern version of attachment theory which they call 'regulation theory'. They are suggesting that an implicit self-system, located in the right hemisphere of the brain and evolving in the preverbal stages of development, serves as the biological substrate of the dynamic unconscious and is centrally involved in 'maintaining a coherent, continuous and unified sense of self' (Devinsky, 2000, cited in Schore and Schore, 2008, p. 12). In the framework of attachment theory, applicable to both humans and dogs, the parent-child relationship influences subsequent development, becoming a key determinant in the offspring's socio-emotional regulation and adaptation. The regulation theory hypothesises that the implicit self-system is in constant interactive regulation, from the early phases of development, through unconscious/implicit emotional transactions with the primary caregiver.

It is yet unclear to what extent can dogs unconsciously represent complex social and interpersonal patterns. But their fundamental homogeneity with humans in this area is clear. Dogs attach to their caretakers and later to other important (sometimes human) figures in their life. They can take part in mutual emotional regulation, and probably have a corresponding implicit self-system, which is always on the look-out for emotional cues in others. Their patterns of relating are reflections of past relationships and they are susceptible to the reactivation of past traumatic experiences via environmental and interpersonal priming. In short, dogs have an inner world of object-relations which inter-permeates their ongoing relations with other organisms, within a context of constant emotional regulation. These findings open the road for us to explore their intrapsychic world using the same language and concepts we use to understand the human psyche.

Mirror neurons and the regulation theory

The neural networks we call mirror systems are situated in certain areas in the pre-motor cortex and take part in coordinating affective states, intents and actions. One of their tasks is to respond to external events, which are related to the actions and intents of other organisms. When someone does something in our field of vision these networks create internal models of the said gesture, via neuronal patterns. Then, other areas in the brain are activated inducing a matching internal state, including a mental intent, a physical affective state and an inclination for action, that mimic the intent, affect and action of the other. It is a kind of a 'mirror game' where you copy the other's movements and emotional cues, only subliminally. Mostly, especially in humans, these mental-physical states are then monitored and constrained through inhibitory circuits and the activation of higher-level processing and decision-making parts of the brain, for the purpose of eliciting a more adaptable behavioral response (Wolf, Gales, Shane and Shane, 2001).

Science always struggled to explain the neuro-biological stratum that enables the movement from the representation of the world of objects to that of the world of subjects, and which forms the platform for our social behavior. The discovery of mirror neurons finally exposed the cerebral particle that functions as the link between subjects. That link whose function makes possible the kind of phenomena that psychoanalysis refers to as unconscious processes, such as Empathy, Mirroring and Projective Identification. Schermer (2010) claims that

> in the world of mirror neurons and mirror systems, individuals attune to one another and represent themselves in and through each other, challenging the premise that minds function in relative isolation. Contrary to the traditional Cartesian dualism separating mind from the body and the material world, mirror systems are distinctly relational, forming a possible linkage among embodied selves, suggesting that, by extension, the mind/brain may be inherently social and intimately linked to its environment and group context (p. 489).

So then, the mirror systems in the brain are an organ specialized in sensing and communicating in the social world, channeling a transpersonal net of interconnected individuals that some refer to as a group mind, or a social matrix (Foulkes, 1973).

A wide research points to mirror neurons as the prime suspect in underlying imitation behaviors in animals, which have a crucial part in the offspring's socialisation and maturation. Mirror neurons were found in monkeys and in some species of songbirds. There is good reason to assume that wherever social behaviors such as imitation and parent-offspring relations exist, mirror neurons will be, especially within social domesticated mammals, such as dogs.

Here is a short example of how mirror systems may work in dogs. I often observe Shula and other dogs in the park approaching each other, each in their own unique ways, sniffing, staring and circling around to assess whether it is safe to get together and play. Shula is a black coated medium size shepherd. She is usually good hearted, but her life has taught her that other dogs can present dangers sometimes. So, she is always a little edgy with new dogs. Sometimes, when the other dog is smaller and/or aggressive and insecure, an instant fight might erupt. In the first fractions of a second, when it starts, it's like a quick chain reaction, where both animals respond to and imitate the other's affective arousal and body language, switching instantly from a calm disposition into a violent one. Supposedly, each party's mirror systems encode and mirror the other's mental and affective state, activating in both the RAGE affective system and inducing a fight mode of behavior.

The relational/social BrainMind

I think that in considering the role and function of mirror systems, we get an idea of the social nature of the BrainMind in mammals, such as dogs. The combined term 'BrainMind' (Panskepp, 2011) reflects the view that mental processes and internal experiences are linked to neural functioning without prioritising either of the two aspects. According to Panskepp (2012), 'the BrainMind is an evolved organ, the only one in the body where evolutionary progressions remain engraved at neuroanatomical, neurochemical, and functional levels' (p. 7). And I would add that it is equally an organ of the self, carrying in it the traces of the evolutionary progressions of relational capacities. In importing the notion of BrainMind, I am underscoring the proposition that relationality is inherent in the genetically determined basic structure and function of both the mental and the neuro-biological realms in all mammals. Mirror neurons may be unique in embodying the elusive connection of mind and body and of self and other.

The last piece of the puzzle is the fact, commonly known and now supported by research, that interpersonal processes that are intermediated by mirror neurons take place between species as well as within them. This has been known since the discovery of mirror neurons, when researchers realised to their surprise that the neuron they were monitoring in a Macaque monkey fired in response to it seeing a human making a specific gesture (Schermer, 2010). Parrots and monkeys have earned a reputation as imitators, although they are certainly not the only species who would willingly participate in such a back and forth interaction with humans. Everyone who owns a cat or a dog has probably many stories to tell about how they play the 'mirror game' with their pet, not unlike parents who play with their toddlers by imitating each other's sounds and movements. I believe mirror neurons facilitate implicit affective transactions beginning with the first proto conversations with neonates.

Dogs in therapy – a summary

What we have here then is a model of a dog with a primary biological self, collected from a constant shifting through affective emotional states, a sense of subjectivity, a consciousness and a social Brain/Mind, constantly connected with and mutually affecting others, including human subjects. A creature who can take part in interpersonal relations has the cerebral equipment to be conscious and empathic, and who can participate in relational processes such as mirroring and projective identification (Roitman, 2019). It may even be that projective identification (or parts of it) is a basic element in the ongoing affective communication between all mammals, as it is said to be in humans (Ogden, 1979).

Dogs are very common as pets and are probably the most prevalent therapeutic animal. These facts are surely related, as many therapists have, or have had dogs as companions at some point in their lives. The changes that *Canine Familiaris* have gone through during their long domestication process and the socialisation of the individual dog in its human surrounding mould the personality of most dogs into something very human-like. Some say that millennia of artificial selection resulted in genetic changes in dogs, favouring socialisation with humans as if they were conspecifics (Topal, Miklosi, Csanyi and Doka, 1998). Most dogs are, in a way, adopted children. They are separated from their mother and siblings at a very early age, in incomprehensible circumstances as far as they are concerned, and are placed in adoptive families and foster homes. This early separation experience is surely encoded within their working-models, later to influence their relationship with their human caretakers and families. Dogs who live with humans learn to read human gestures and affective signals and adapt their regulatory functions to the human implicit affective communication vocabulary. In dogs' working models, human representations and interactive patterns with humans must occupy a considerable part.

In the second part of the chapter, I will present some clinical moments from the psychotherapy of a child, in which my dog, Shula, was a central participant. In discussing these vignettes, I will demonstrate how the theoretical considerations that I have elaborated so far enable us to incorporate a deeper understanding of the dog's side of the relational processes that transpire. With this understanding, new possibilities will emerge to clinically assess what is going on in the therapeutic process, thereby enriching our options as therapists to think and respond in ways that enhance the therapeutic value of our work.

Part II: Clinical and technical applications: the case of Kori and Shula playing ball

Kori is an eleven-year-old oppositional and avoidant child, who is overly concerned with his physical health and seems to underestimate his resilience.

He avoids taking risks and applying effort, shies away from social activities, and therefore is left socially isolated and academically regressed. His general demeanor is gloomy and withdrawn. In the first months of therapy, we spent most of our time in the backyard outside the therapy room. Kori would hesitantly try various physical challenges, like trimming grass with hedge shears and climbing trees, and gradually became more confident with his physicality.

Shula was always around, watching us, keeping close to me and usually ready to join in whenever one of us called her. At first, Kori would acknowledge her without making contact, or would comment on what he thinks her mood was. After some time, he began touching her fleetingly, with my close presence as intermediator, and was very wary of the area around her mouth and specifically her teeth. Then he started to play with her. A few months into therapy he invented a game: he would hold her favourite ball in his hand, waving it back and forth as if he is about to throw it for her to fetch. Shula would get excited and jump up and down, in response to which Kori would sometimes laugh with pleasure. Then he would make a strong throwing motion while saying 'Shula, go fetch', but wouldn't release the ball. Shula would jolt in the direction of the anticipated flight of the ball, but instantly realizing that the ball is nowhere in that vicinity she would stop short, turn back and look at us confused, to Kori's clear pleasure. Kori would then call her and show her the ball in his hand. At first, Shula would hesitate, as if weighing whether to withdraw, but most of the time she would comply and re-engage back in the game. But, in seeing her approaching, Kori would recoil in instant fear or hide behind my back, asking me to hold her. Only after restoring his courage, he would start over and repeat the whole procedure from the top.

In this game that Kori played with Shula, both have undergone several shifts in self-states (Bromberg, 1996). I think that for Kori it was these shifts in Shula's affective-emotional states that were the interesting aspect of the game. In the language of affective neuroscience, we can speculatively track the changes in the affective arousal in both participants of this interaction. To my mind, Kori's gestures with the ball were a trigger for the activation of the PLAY system in Shula, eliciting corresponding affective-emotional reactions in her mind and body, that could be related to the human emotions of joy, excitement and playfulness. Her behavior expressed these emotions and her willingness to be part of the game. For the hesitant and restrained boy, seeing her jumping excitedly in the air in such an overt manner seemed to elicit a quite similar, albeit uncommon, affective-emotional state and behaviour. In the realm of mirror neurons, this mutual affective regulation can be explained by the activation of each participant's mirror systems, which generated an inner affective-intentional-behavioral state, mirroring that of its counterpart. Thus, a bi-directional communication was taking place, co-creating an interpersonal field, an 'analytic third' (Ogden, 1994), exuberant and lively with the anticipation for mutual play. In the analytic relationship between Kori and myself it was only many months later until we achieved such a place together.

But the fun was not to last long. The sudden change in the anticipated course of the game, when Shula's flow was arrested and she found herself chasing nothing, also changed abruptly her emotional experience. Shula's reaction seemed to express surprise and confusion. At the level of affective systems, we could speak of the disappointment resulting from the activation of a state of SEEKING without supplying the ensuing reward. Kori's response to that was, most surprisingly, a show of glee and satisfaction. More complex emotions that I saw as manifestations of the inner conflicts and dramas that were reenacted for him through this interaction. It was clear that making Shula feel this way was eliciting ambivalent feelings in Kori. I thought I saw in him a sense of power and mastery that made him feel mighty and happy, along with a hostile-aggressive part, which accounted for his glee and satisfaction facing Shula's distress. But I could also detect feelings of shame and probably remorse and self-condemnation, which were responsible for the fear (of retaliation) that arose later when Shula began making her way back towards us.

In fact, Shula now would always come back to me, not to Kori. The boy at that stage was usually hiding behind me, and his stare and body language expressed fear and avoidance. I think that both at that point were in a distressed PANIC state, seeking comfort. I believe that in the first instants after the dramatic twist in the game, seconds after Shula hit the brakes, there was a moment when they exchanged looks and affective states, via the mirror systems in each, and this was the moment of change in the general atmosphere of the interaction. A mood-contagion was taking effect again, influencing them simultaneously.

So now here I was, a wailing wall[3] to both, one behind my back and one at my front. At that point, for the game to recommence, my emotional participation was needed. Each time this happened, I found myself intervening as if being activated to resolve and dissolve the interpersonal block that has appeared between them. I would then caress Shula, talk calmly and reassuringly to her while explaining to Kori what I think he and Shula felt at that moment and that there was nothing for him to fear. I'm sure that my tone and affective state played a part in restoring, in both child and dog, confidence, curiosity and the motivation to play. Here again, I assume that it was with the mediation of the mirror neurons in all of us, that this group regulation was made possible, and the game resumed.

Intrapsychic, intersubjective and relational perspectives alternate

Watching Kori's way of playing the ball game with Shula made me think of the roles they both played as representing his experience with his father, a somber man with anxious and hypochondriac characteristics. Whenever Kori would show enthusiasm, his father would react in an over-protective manner, restraining him while pointing to possible hazards and physical dangers. On the current level, in his game with Shula, it was as if a bigger force from within was restraining Kori, preventing him again and again from following through with his intention to throw the ball. And every time, when that happened, Shula would react with surprise and confusion, possibly reflecting for Kori his self-state in reaction to his father's protective grip. Kori's show of glee and satisfaction was, in my mind, a sign of his identification with the father's need for control and his disavowed hostility and envy at the child's spontaneity, self-confidence and playfulness.

In his wish to repeat the pleasurable experience and maintain his control over the dog, Kori would tempt her then back into another session of his tantalizing game. But now, watching her depleted of her former energetic state, he felt he had to revive her into a playful mood again. Waving the ball at her and calling her were gestures that I could again connect in my mind to his parents, especially his mother, who relentlessly encouraged and sweet-talked him, trying desperately to make him get up, get dressed, go to school, join social activities and do his homework.

But what struck me as most curious was his emerging anxiety, as Shula was coming towards us. He clearly had felt in danger. As I mentioned earlier, I thought that for him, it was his projected sadistic urge that was now deposited in Shula and was coming after him. An overwhelming fear, arising from the activation of some early experience, had now overshadowed his ability to read Shula's affective state correctly, using his regular sensors. What he saw at that moment was not a disappointed dog, looking for a comforting touch and eager to reengage in play. In his eyes, she was a predator with huge teeth coming at him with vengeful rage. A part of himself, a disavowed self-state, was too scary to express or even acknowledge.

Veering our attention now to Shula, let us see what more we can say about her intrapsychic experience. Here is her history in brief: Shula was first adopted as a pup, separated from her litter and her mother at the age of two months. She lived with a young woman in an urban flat but had to be given away after the landlord forbade the owner to keep animals in the apartment. I took her in when she was six months old. When she joined my family, we had a newborn girl, who is now 8 and has a brother aged 6. Shula spends most of her time in the yard, where she has her kennel and lots of space, but likes to lie around inside the house when we let her. While I am in my clinic, which is also a part of the house, she usually hangs outside my therapy-room door, in the waiting hall, until invited to join the session.

Thinking about her early days, Shula was taken from her mother at an age when pups are usually weaned and reach independence in all their bodily functions, and their main efforts are mobilized to playing and socializing. But Shula couldn't stay longer with her siblings. I don't know much about her time in the city and her relationship with her first owner, nor about how she reacted to her two separation experiences. Since I adopted her, she hasn't had much playtime with other dogs. Most of the time she was alone in the big yard, and sometimes with us who were busy with our own babies and our human affairs. In the house next door lives a family with a pack of three or four dogs. It's their habit to bark violently at anyone coming close to their fence. They are especially fond of barking at other dogs. In her first years with us Shula would frequently get enraged and launch at them, from her side of the fence, barking and growling with bare teeth and bristled mane.

I think that these selected facts from her life story are important because they account for some personality traits in Shula that are relevant for the analysis of her interpersonal patterns. As I have mentioned in the first example with Shula, she tends to be quite edgy around other dogs and I have noticed that even if the first encounter goes well, she doesn't really know how to play with them. Her playstyle is too rough for most dogs, and she quickly loses interest. With humans, she learned to allow kids to be around her and touch her (this is something that I took the time to teach her) but seems quite indifferent towards them and prefers to get the attention of adults. In a way, she is a bit like an only child who never learned how to get along with his peers and only strives to please and get attention and affection from grown-ups. Someone who other kids quickly grow tired of, and who grows to be a loner.

Knowing her character, I had anticipated that Shula would be happy to join Kori in a game of 'fetch the ball', which she knew very well, and would enjoy the satisfaction of accomplishing what her human counterpart would ask of her. But when the game took an unexpected turn Shula didn't know anymore what was expected of her and got confused. She didn't immediately 'play along' with the new rules, as some dogs might have done, but lost her spirit and redirected herself to me, the authority and parental figure, for guidance.

While writing these lines, it comes to my mind that there is something in Shula that reminds me of Kori in those first months of therapy. Albeit for different reasons, both were children who couldn't play and whose social adjustment was impaired. Both had been over-concerned with their relations with adults and authority figures to be bothered with their peers.

Where was I when all this was going on? I must admit that I felt very uncomfortable with Kori's behaviour towards Shula. I decided to bite my tongue though because I trusted Shula to withdraw from the game if it would become too frustrating for her. I've seen her do that many times before. So, I didn't discourage Kori from resuming the game a few times, and at some point, he would just let go and move on to something else, mostly not involving Shula. Or, she would just tire and not come back for another round.

My discomfort was partly due to my empathy with Shula. I think that a hostile angry self-state in me was resonating a denied part of Kori's affective-emotional state. I saw Kori at that moment as a perpetrator and Shula as a victim. This created a conflict with my warm and caring feelings towards the boy. By allowing him to engage with Shula without my interruption I was modeling a way to contain the conflict and the tension, while resisting the urge to take control and ward off my anxiety by restraining him, thereby preventing him from exploring an important, albeit unacknowledged, self-state. At the same time, I had to remain watchful and avoid another urge to look away. It was up to me to stay emotionally open to what was going on inside myself and inside Kori and Shula and be ready to intervene at the right time. In this way, I served both as a witness and as a parental guardian, waiting for my cue to step in and help process excess stress and anxiety in the matrix when needed to.

In Benjamin's terms (2004), I was introducing the 'third in the one' to the matrix, an attitude that reflected my recognition of the other's subjectivity and trust in the process of maturation and growth through interpersonal relations. I believe that my presence was helpful in moving the matrix towards becoming more intersubjective. In tuning my empathy towards the others in the field and making myself accessible to them emotionally, when they needed me to, I was making room for an exchange of feelings and self-states, thereby facilitating affective communication (Maroda, 2002). In addressing Shula's emotional state, acknowledging it out loud and offering compassion I was assisting Kori, so I believe, to recognize her as a subject and gain a better understanding of the reality of his relationship with her. By reflecting on what I thought he was experiencing and by soothing his fears I was making him know that I recognize his subjectivity as well. I suggest that, to some degree, the same is true with Shula. That for her, looking at me looking at her empathically, hearing my words, seeing my facial expressions and feeling my hand gestures responding to her subjectivity, was a vitalising experience that reawakened and rewarded her capacity to see us humans as subjects. I became a witness to both their intrapsychic realities and helped pave the road for them to meet each other anew within an intersubjective matrix.

This short but rich interaction, involving the three of us, was made of many tiny relational moments, all channeled through the activation and mediation of our primary affective systems, our implicit memories and relational patterns, and our neuronal mirror systems. I believe one can show how relational processes, such as empathy, mirroring and projective identification, were also involved. In terms of self-states, it is an example of the way an animal in therapy can help the emergence of disavowed self-states and assist, with the aid of the therapist, in recognizing them and processing them. As Bromberg (1996) and others suggest, the renegotiation and integration of disassociated self-states are one of the desired outcomes of therapy. One can also see here how mutual regulation and affective contagion were involved and how they were helpful in the development and honing of interpersonal skills and in the creation and maintenance of transitional space in the analytic session.

Changing over time – Kori dubs Shula a superhero

About two and a half years later Kori came one day to therapy in a very good mood. It was summer by then, too hot to be outside. Before entering the room, he stopped next to Shula, sprawled on the waiting room floor, and gave her a long hug. Shula seemed happy to see him and licked his face, her tail thumping the floor rhythmically. He then came in and called her to join us. Shula got up heavily, stretched and followed him. They spent long moments playing together during that session. At some point Kori challenged her to guess in which of his closed fists he was hiding a tissue paper. Shula was clearly trying to figure out what was the game about, and sniffed his hands randomly, which was a sign for him to open his palms and declare her success or failure. Interestingly, and to Kori's delight, it seemed that after a few trials, Shula's success rate increased. Had she actually gotten better at finding where the paper was hidden? Or maybe it was Kori who had made it easier for her, unconsciously moving the hand with the prize closer to her nose? At another moment I noticed that while telling me about some events from his life Kori had his hand resting casually on Shula's back. Later in the session he took another tissue paper and stuffed its edge around Shula's neck-collar to make it into a cape and tried to blow some air to make it flutter, saying that Shula is a superhero. I was impressed by how permissive and playful Shula was. She is not the kind of dog that kids can climb on top of and pull her ear. But at that moment it was obvious that she enjoyed his touch and was rubbing herself against his body and licking him when he let her. I felt warm emotions watching this intimate moment between them.

I've included this second moment in Kori and Shula's relationship to offer another perspective of the consequences of the integration of dogs in therapy. We are accustomed to speaking about the long-term effect of the therapeutic relationship between a patient and an analyst. Discussions addressing transference, enactment and other relational processes stress the importance of time in the resolution of therapeutic challenges and interpersonal entanglements. All relational analysts would agree that a successful treatment is one in which the therapist changes as well, in relation to the change in the patient. According to the regulation theory, we are in a constant state of change. Change, within a social context, is an inevitable part of being in a relationship. Dogs are relational beings, as we have seen, and are not excluded from this rule.

Both Shula and Kori have changed during these two and a half years, regardless of their relationship within the therapeutic setting. But it is my belief and clinical impression that their time together has made an impact on both their persons and on their working-models, in a way that contributed to them in other social circles and interpersonal encounters. The theoretical model that was presented in the first part of this chapter implies that there exists, at least potentially, a large measure of plasticity in the relational capacities of both the dog and the human self. The ongoing relationship of the patient with the dog, quite like the one he has with his analyst, has the potential to bring about deep changes to all. In Kori's therapy, Shula has become an important figure for him. He has found in her a friend and partner for play, an attachment figure whose presence offers comfort and a secure base to go back to after distressing experiences, a transitional object to destroy and revive in fantasy at will and a reflection of some parts of himself that were made accessible and more tolerable as their connection grew stronger and more intimate. A similar change was observable in Shula, who became more relaxed and amiable in his presence, showing clear signs of affection and an increased ability to tolerate ambiguity and physical intimacy. I think Kori has become like a brother to her, thus facilitating the development of her capacity to play.

Much more can be said about this second vignette and about the symbolic meaning of the interactions therein, and the neuro-psychological and relational mechanisms that took part in their making. But I will let it speak for itself and move on to some concluding notes.

Part III: Technical considerations and summary

The theory that I have presented on animal relationality and its implications on dog- assisted psychotherapy has, to my mind, some technical derivatives. As it may have struck the reader in my earlier discussions, it demands that the therapist adopt a multi-focal stance which holds in mind simultaneously three very different perspectives. The first would be the physical level, where phenomena such as emotional-affective activation and affective resonance via mirror systems occur. Bearing in mind these relational-neurological mechanisms helps to understand the moment-to-moment dynamics of the dog-patient interactions in the here-and-now. It can give us tools to decipher the mutual influence that the two exert on each other, which enables processes of mutual regulation and implicit, or unconscious, communication. The second level of awareness is the relational level, in which two subjectivities meet, each with its own inner world of feelings, working models, fears and expectations. This is a perspective focusing on the interpersonal encounter where both subjects reenact and renegotiate interpersonal patterns and mutually struggle to integrate disowned parts of their selves and to improve their capacity to play. The third and last level is the wider angle that takes into account group phenomena, relating to the multiple interactions between all participants, including the therapist. I will elaborate on this axis of the theoretical model in the next chapter.

At any given moment in the session, it is our job to assess what is going on in all three levels and be ready to intervene in a way that helps resolve interpersonal deadlocks and removes obstacles from a free-flowing interaction. We should strive to identify negative affective states and moments of reactivation / reenactment of traumatic implicit memories and working models, and act in ways that restore a positive interpersonal atmosphere, to allow the continuous working through of these toxic moments. In the vignette above, depicting the ballgame between Shula and Kori, I described such a moment and the way I found to bridge the hostility and alienation that immerged between them, in hope of reengaging them to find better ways to play together.

It is of crucial importance that the therapist be comfortable with the dog and experienced in handling dogs in distress, just as he is necessarily trained in helping humans in hurt. The relational model here described advocates treating the animal as an essentially similar subject, whose affective state and regulation is equally important to address, as are those of the child patient.

It is also important to remember that the therapeutic setting is not just the place where the treatment is happening but also a dynamic and interactive living presence (Roitman and Kassirer-Izraeli, 2013). Adding a dog to a one-on-one classical setting increases the levels of responsivity and interactivity of the setting. In our function as dynamic administrators and (parental) managers of the setting, we must pay attention to the relationship of the patient with the setting. The dog in therapy is also a part of that setting and can be of positive or negative influence on the patient's sense of security and to his capacity to surrender (Ghent, 1990) to the therapeutic process. In my practice, I can recall numerous occasions in which I decided to remove Shula's presence from the session, and even from the road leading from the exterior gate to the waiting room. These were cases in which my impression was that her mere presence would result in excess anxiety in the patient I was about to see. At times, a dog in the therapeutic space can make the setting too menacing for the child.

Another technical aspect is concerned with the implication of treating the dog as a subject. The principle of 'the animal as a subject' is both the ethical and the theoretical backdrop of the theoretical model I am proposing. Using this model means to make room for the dog's subjectivity in the therapeutic discourse. Taking this idea to the technical level, treating the dog as a subject means addressing it in similar ways that we address a human subject. It is my belief and experience that when we relate to dogs as subjects, in words, gestures and touch, it awakens their sense of subjectivity and motivates them to engage in intersubjective interactions. The attitude of the therapist here is of utmost importance, as a model to both child and dog in creating the right 'rules of engagement' for the therapeutic encounter.

Summary

The relational approach to dog-assisted child psychotherapy proposed here is very brief with general guidelines. Much more needs to be explored and elaborated. As I have pointed out, the psychoanalytical literature and the papers addressing the principles of the psychotherapeutic technique have so far done little to include the implications of a theory on the human-animal connection to the psychotherapy of children. This is part of a general trend that ignores the study of the human-animal relationships in the psychological sciences (Melson, 2002). For example, I think that we need to develop a better understanding of the unconscious processes between humans and animals. (Roitman, 2019). Exploring these processes, in the context of the neuroscientific-relational perspective, can clear up fundamental aspects of the effects of AAP and even illuminate some unvisited aspects of unconscious processes between humans.

On an ethical note, I believe that seeing and treating the dog as a subject is a first and important step in advancing a more equal approach to animals. This is part of a social duty that we all carry, as moral human beings and as therapists. The ethical point of view on the incorporation of animals in the treatment of humans also deserves more attention and elaboration.

What is suggested in the first part of this chapter and illustrated in the second is part of a three-axis theoretical model to animal-assisted-psychotherapy, with emphasis on the participation of a dog in a one-on-one therapy of a child patient. In this chapter, the focus was on the neuropsychological and the relational axes. The third axis will be formulated in the next chapter, presenting a group approach to AAP. It is this writer's opinion that the three-axis model potentially encompasses all the fundamental aspects involved in AAP and is necessary for therapists who wish to muster the relational potential of animals to the benefit of the psychotherapeutic endeavor, be it incidentally or as a method of treatment.

Notes

1 I am not ignoring the immense differences between humans and animals, pointed out by Darwin himself and many others (see for example Kolstad, 2013), which come from the fact that the human environment has become more cultural and social than natural. My point is only that these differences have not succeeded in effacing the evolutionary continuity and the basic functional homology between humans and animals.

2 Very relevant here is the 'Cambridge Declaration on Consciousness', in which leading scientists declared in 2012 that '…the weight of evidence indicates that humans are not unique in possessing the neurological substrates that generate consciousness.' The Cambridge Declaration on Consciousness was written by Philip Low and edited by Jaak Panksepp, Diana Reiss, David Edelman, Bruno Van Swinderen, Philip Low and Christof Koch. The Declaration was publicly proclaimed in Cambridge, UK, on July 7, 2012, at the Francis Crick Memorial Conference on Consciousness in Human and non-Human Animals, at Churchill College, University of Cambridge, by Low, Edelman and Koch.

3 According to the Merriam-Webster dictionary: (1) Capitalised: A surviving section of the wall which in ancient times formed a part of the enclosure of Herod's temple near the Holy of Holies in Jerusalem, and at which Jews traditionally gather for prayer and religious lament. (2) A source of comfort and consolation in misfortune.

References

Asma, S. T. and Greif, T. (2012) Affective neuroscience and the philosophy of self. In the philosophical implications of affective neuroscience. *Journal of Consciousness Studies*, 19(3–4), pp. 28–36.

Benjamin, J. (2004) Beyond doer and done to: An intersubjective view of thirdness. *Psychoanalytic Quarterly*, 73(1), pp. 5–46.

Berger, J. (1980) *About looking.* New York: Pantheon.

Bowlby, J. (1969) *Attachment and loss*, Vol. 1. Attachment. New York: Basic Books.

Bromberg, P. M. (1996) Standing in the spaces: The multiplicity of self and the psychoanalytic relationship. *Contemporary Psychoanalysis*, 32(4), pp. 509–535.

Damasio, A. (1999) *The feeling of what happens: Body, emotion and the making of consciousness.* San Diego, CA: Harcourt Brace.

Darwin, C. (1871) *The descent of man and selection in relation to sex.* Princeton, NJ: Princeton University Press.

Foulkes, S. H. (1973) The group as matrix of the individual's mental life. In: L. R. Wolberg and E. K. Schwartz (Eds.), *Group therapy: An overview.* New York: Intercontinental Medical Book Corporation, pp. 223–233.

Freud, S. (1917) A difficulty in the path of psycho-analysis. The standard edition *of the complete psychological works of Sigmund Freud*, Volume 27 (1917–1919).

Ghent, E. (1990) Masochism, submission, surrender: Masochism as a perversion of surrender. *Contemporary Psychoanalysis*, 26(1), pp. 108–136.

Graf, P. and Schacter, D. L. (1985) Implicit and explicit memory for new associations in normal and amnesic subjects. *Journal of Experimental Psychology: Learning, Memory, and Cognition*, 11(3), pp. 501–518.

Grossman, D. (2004) *Someone to run with.* New York: Farrar, Straus & Giroux.

Harari, Y. N. (2014) *Sapiens: A brief history of humankind.* London: Vintage.

Horn, L., Huber, L. and Range, F. (2013) The importance of the secure base effect for domestic dogs: Evidence from a manipulative problem-solving task. *PLoS One*, 8(5), e65296. doi:10.1371/journal.pone.0065296.

Kolstad, A. (2013) Human psychological characteristics versus animal characteristics. *Psychology*, 4(5), pp. 488–493. doi:10.4236/psych.2013.45069.

Low, P. (2012) The Cambridge declaration on consciousness [Online]. Available at: http://fcmconference.org/img/CambridgeDeclarationOnConsciousness.pdf. Accessed October 2, 2019.

Maroda, K. (2002) No place to hide: Affectivity, the unconscious, and the development of relational technique. *Contemporary Psychoanalysis*, 38(1), pp. 101–120.

Melson, G. F. (2002) Psychology and the study of human-animal relationships. *Society & Animals*, 10(4), pp. 347–352.

Myers, G. (1998) *Children and animals: Social development and our connection to other species.* Boulder, CO: Westview.

Ogden, T. H. (1979) On projective identification. *International Journal of Psychoanalysis*, 60(3), pp. 357–373.

Ogden, T. H. (1994) *Subjects of analysis.* New York: Aronson.

Panksepp, J. (2001). The neuro-evolutionary cusp between emotions and cognitions. *Evolution and Cognition*, 7(2), pp. 141–163.

Panksepp, J. (2011) Cross-species affective neuroscience decoding of the primal affective experiences of humans and related animals. *PLoS One*, 6(9), e21236. doi:10.1371/journal.pone.0021236.

Panksepp, J. (2012) A synopsis of affective neuroscience: Naturalizing the mammalian brain. In the philosophical implications of affective neuroscience. *Journal of Consciousness Studies*, 19(3–4), pp. 6–18.

Rajecki, D. W., Lamb, M. E. and Obmascher, P. (1978) Toward a general theory of infantile attachment: A comparative review of aspects of the social bond. *Behavioral and Rain Sciences*, 1(3), pp. 417–436.

Roitman, D. (2019) People, animals and unconscious interpersonal processes: Inter-subjectivity in the human-animal bond in animal-assisted-therapy and beyond it [Online]. Available at: https://www.hebpsy.net/articles.asp?id=3797. Accessed August 3, 2019 [In Hebrew].

Roitman, D. and Kassirer-Izraeli, H. (2013) The therapeutic setting as a living presence: Considerations on child psychotherapy in a therapy zoo. *Sihot*, 28(1), pp. 67–76 [In Hebrew].

Schacter, D. L. (1987) Implicit memory: History and current status. *Journal of Experimental Psychology: Learning, Memory, and Cognition*, 13(3), pp. 501–518.

Schermer, V. L. (2010) Mirror neurons: Their implications for group psychotherapy. *International Journal of Group Psychotherapy*, 60(4), pp. 487–513.

Schore, A. L. (2000) Attachment and the regulation of the right brain. *Attachment & Human Development*, 2(1), pp. 23–47.

Schore, A. N. (1994) *Affect regulation and the origin of the self*. Mahweh, NJ: Erlbaum.

Schore, A. N. (2005) Attachment, affect regulation, and the developing right brain: Linking developmental neuroscience to pediatrics. *Pediatrics in Review*, 26(6), pp. 204–211.

Schore, J. R. and Schore, A. L. (2008) Modern attachment theory: The central role of affect regulation in development and treatment. *Journal of Clinical Social Work*, 36(1), pp. 9–20.

Solms, M. (2013) The conscious id. *Journal of Neuropsychoanalysis*, 15(1), pp. 5–19.

Topal, J., Miklosi, A., Csanyi, V. and Doka, A. (1998) Attachment behavior in dogs (*Canis Familiaris*): A new application of Ainsworth's (1969) strange situation test. *Journal of Comparative Psychology*, 112(3), pp. 219–229.

Wolf, N. S., Gales, M. E., Shane, E. and Shane, M. (2001) The developmental trajectory from amodal perception to empathy and communication: The role of mirror neurons in this process. *Psychoanalytic Enquiry*, 21(1), pp. 94–112.

6 A journey inside Noah's ark

A group analytic theory of child psychotherapy in a therapy zoo

Dor Roitman

So is written in Genesis, Chapter 6:

> **(6)**[18] But with thee will I establish my covenant; and thou shalt come into the ark, thou, and thy sons, and thy wife, and thy sons' wives with thee.[19] And of every living thing of all flesh, two of every sort shalt thou bring into the ark, to keep them alive with thee; they shall be male and female.[20] Of fowls after their kind, and of cattle after their kind, of every creeping thing of the earth after his kind, two of every sort shall come unto thee, to keep them alive.[21] And take thou unto thee of all food that is eaten, and thou shalt gather it to thee; and it shall be for food for thee, and for them.[22] Thus did Noah; according to all that God commanded him, so did he.

The notion of Noah's Ark came to me as I was thinking of a title for this chapter. It struck me that no word is said in the scriptures about what happened inside the ark during the deluge and the flood, which lasted a year and eleven days.[1] The biblical myth depicts the great flood as a punishment visited upon humankind for their sins vis-à-vis God and their fellow humans. The sins are moral in nature. It is thus a text which deals with moral purge and reconstitution. Into the ark went Noah, chosen by his God, and with him his family and a selection of animals. I like the idea that the Ark can also represent the analytic space. Firmly defined and secluded from the outer world, it is a space to which a person can withdraw from life's marathon, from the demands and stressors of earthly mundane business and engage in self-development, in a search for inner resources and in the appeasement of moral conflicts. Contemporary approaches focus on the patient's experience of emotional isolation and psychic stagnation, and on the task of finding one's place in the world within the interpersonal fabric of one's community[2]. Therefore, the patient is not alone in his journey. The analyst is there with him as an Other, a subject who makes herself available for emotional involvement. The relational school, unifying under its wings a variety of psychoanalytic approaches, sees the meeting of subjects, or minds, in therapy as both the spark that ignites and the engine that pushes the therapeutic process forward.

Clearly, the biblical narrator locates Noah as the protagonist, in relation to which all other characters, human and non-human, remain in the background. The tension in the story revolves around Noah's relationship with God. The only hint as to Noah's state of mind is given in Chapter 6 verse 22: 'Thus did Noah; according to all that God commanded him, so did he'. This narrow behavioural description is so tight that we can virtually feel Noah's awful terror and trepidation in the presence of the Almighty, the supreme authority who has chosen and who commands him. At the same time, the scriptures leave no doubt that this journey is about family, community and the survival and prosperity of all those 'wherein is the breath of life' (Chapter 7, Verse 15). God makes a point of populating the ark with couples, from Noah and his wife, his sons and their wives, to the rest of the animals, always male with female, priming the reader to think of them as couples, fathers and mothers, procreative units, all selected and personally separated from the rest of their kind. And there is another being present in this journey, although in a more subtle, decentred way. It is God himself, always watching but rarely intervening, in a voice that probably only Noah can hear. In a wider context, God's presence is strongly felt by all, of course. He is the one who architected the ark, broke up 'all the fountains of the great deep' (Chapter 7, Verse 11) and is the initiator and orchestrator of the whole journey.

The intimate relationship between God and Noah, which includes a deep scrutiny into the latter's soul, is backboned by an alliance which God drafted and brought to Noah to sign. In my interpretation, Noah is in the role of the patient, ready to act first and understand later, for the sake of saving his soul and his community. God, then, is in the role of the animal-assisted therapist, aware of the vital importance of the presence of animals in the healing and survival of the human race. Being a group analyst as well, he can appreciate the intra-psychic, inter-personal and social impact of group processes, and knows how to marginalise himself and minimise his authoritative presence, once the ark has been set on its course, to allow for a maximum degree of freedom in the contact and communication among the other participants. According to this interpretation, God intended the ark to be a floating therapy zoo, meant to treat the sick human race through Noah, its chosen representative, via group-analytic animal-assisted therapy. A method more commonly referred to as Animal-Assisted Psychotherapy (AAP) in a therapy zoo.

In this chapter I will try to fill in the gap in the scriptures and describe some of what may have taken place inside the ark during its journey. The present chapter aims to offer a group-analytic perspective on the practice of AAP in a therapy zoo. It is also a part of a theoretical project, which tries to draw some preliminary outlines around a three-axis theoretical framework for AAP. The group-analytic axis adds to the neuro-psychoanalytic and the relational axes, presented in Chapter 4. The main body of the present chapter will be divided into a theoretical and a clinical part. First I will discuss the setting of the therapy zoo through the group-analytic perspective, and try to contextualise the psychotherapy of children, within this setting, by using group-analytic concepts and by comparing it to the model of the 'small group' in group-analysis. In the second part, using a case study, I will illustrate and discuss the implications of looking at child-psychotherapy in a therapy zoo through the group-analytic lens.

Part I: child psychotherapy in the therapy zoo: a group analytic exploration

My main line of thought will be as follows: since habitats, or 'niches', in the therapy zoo, are social systems, it is therefore possible to analyse the dynamics therein in terms of the tripartite matrix (Nitzgen and Hopper, 2018; Hopper, 2018), emphasising the primordial socio-biological inheritance, which is an aspect of the foundation matrix (Foulkes, 1973; Bacha, 2019). The communication among individuals in the tripartite matrix is initially understood as operating implicitly, conveying mostly emotional states. Emotions are the basic currency in the transpersonal network of communication and are the embodiment of the social nature of all mammals, avians and arguably, all vertebrates. Within this multifaceted matrix the therapeutic dyad is conceived, born and developed. Embedded in the community of animals, it becomes a part of the matrix and a new phenomenon is created, which can be compared to the small analytic group.

Social animals

S. H. Foulkes founded the group analytic method of group therapy and research out of a deep belief that humans are social beings through and through. He wrote:

> What is inside is outside, the 'social' is not external but very much internal too and penetrates the innermost being of the individual personality. The 'objective' external 'reality' is inseparable from the being, animal or human, and indeed the individual whose world it is and therefore is part of the 'psychological' reality as well (Foulkes, 1973, p. 227).

Stacey (2001) explores this idea by comparing two approaches. In the first, drawing on Brown (1994) and building on object-relations theories, he formulates a view of the individual psyche that emerges in a social context through processes of projection and internalisation, as an 'internal world' consisting of representations of objects (including the self) and relationships between them. This representation system is an action system that lies 'behind' social interactions, motivating and affecting them, while being affected and constantly created by them. The social is also present 'outside' these social interactions, in the norms, values, customs and so on, that impregnate the internalised objects and relationships. This, he says, is how the social is transmitted from one generation to the next. Stacey compares this view to a second approach, which he bases on Mead (1934), who saw the social as an interactive process of meaningful gesturing and signalling between bodies in continuous cycles of cooperation and competition. According to Mead, Mind and Self emerge in social relationships. They are interpersonal processes made up of communicative actions and interactions, rather than entities that can be located within individuals. The individual psyche is then inherently social, being a communicative interaction of a body (the 'I') with itself (the 'me').

Current theories of attachment and regulation, as well as a growing body of neuroscientific findings, provide ample evidence for the natural induction that animals too are social by nature. In the previous chapter, I wrote about the animal self and its relational aspect, drawing on several fields of neurological research. Once we have broken the mental barrier and overcome our resistance to speaking about the relational self in animals, the road is open for us to consider the deep implications of animal sociality. While reading the previous paragraph, the reader may have noticed that in discussing the place of the social in the individual's life, there was no need for the word 'human' or for any of its derivatives. It seems that this discussion is as relevant to animals as it is to humans. The object relations perspective can easily be applied to animals, as discussed in Chapter 4, in connection to what we know about implicit knowledge and about the operation of internal working models in animals. The second perspective echoes the theories, outlined in Chapter 4, about the basic emotional systems, implicit communication and emotional regulation, and about the role of mirror neurons in development and social adjustment.

Lavie (2005), in his paper on the roots of the theory of Group Analysis, elaborates on Foulkes' ideas about socialisation and individuation as two parts of a simultaneous-interdependent process, through which individuals (and social systems such as groups and institutions) develop, within a specific social context. He thereby adheres to Foulkes' conviction, drawing on the work of Norbert Elias, that the individual is not a closed but an 'open system' (Fuchs, 1938). I think that the notion of inter-related individuals, of open systems or social beings, captures the essence not only of how relational psychoanalysis and group analysis see human individuals but also constitutes the cornerstone of the theory of AAP proposed here. Namely, that human and non-human individuals are inherently social and that any grouping of these inter-related open systems will create a potentially transformational context for the individuals within it. Community life in the animal habitat in the therapy zoo, providing that it offers minimal conditions for a safe environment suitable for the animals to live prosperously and interact freely, is an example of such a context.

The matrix in the therapy zoo

Therapy zoos are specified adaptations of menageries and petting zoos. Roitman and Kassirer-Izraeli (2013) have pointed out four elements composing the physical experience in the therapy zoo. These are: (1) A hands-on contact with natural elements and with the rhythm of natural cycles and nature's permanent changing. (2) A variety of possibilities for moving around, between niches and through gates, doors and passageways. (3) An explosion of multi-sensual stimulation. (4) Rich opportunities for interactions with a variety of animals. It is the latter that interests us here. Animals in the therapy zoo are bred and lodged in niches, each designed as a specific habitat to suit a community of individuals of one or more species. These communities qualify as social systems because we can discern the set of variables 'in which a change in any one of them can be explained by changes in one or more of the other variables in the set' (Hopper, 2018, p. 199). If we introduce a new male rabbit into an existing community of rabbits, we will notice changes in the behaviours of other rabbits, as well as a change in the general behaviour of the pack. For instance, a veteran adult male (a buck) may exhibit unusual hostility while a female (a doe) may show signs of excited curiosity. In fact, the whole community will react to the newcomer, mobilizing various subsystems to reach a new systemic equilibrium. One can assess these animal communities through the same dimensions that Hopper (2018) mentions as featuring in all social systems. These are complexity and simplicity (in terms of role differentiation and specialization), cohesion–incohesion, closure–openness, dynamism–static and stability–instability.

Foulkes used the term 'Matrix' to draw attention to the transpersonal network of communication within and among the participants in a group (Foulkes, 1973). Working with groups inspired Foulkes to theorize about a 'supra-personal mental matrix', which is a mental field of operation that includes the individual but also transcends him, and in which all the transpersonal processes occur. 'These processes pass through the individual, though each individual elaborates them and contributes to them and modifies them in his own way. Nevertheless, they go through all the individuals – similar to X-rays in the physical sphere' (p. 229). He realised that thinking just in terms of individual interacting minds wasn't enough to make sense of the enormous complexity of processes, actions and interactions between even two or three parties, let alone explain how they can understand each other and 'to some extent refer to a shared and common sense of what is going on'. He says,

> Instead, I have accepted from the beginning that even this group of total strangers, being of the same species and more narrowly of the same culture, share a fundamental, mental matrix (foundation matrix). To this their closer acquaintance and their intimate exchanges add consistently, so that they also form a current, ever-moving, ever-developing dynamic matrix (p. 228).

Nitzgen and Hopper (2018) suggest a tripartite formulation of the matrix, in which the personal-matrix is added to the foundation-matrix and the dynamic-matrix, the personal matrix being the mental field of interacting processes composing the individual mind. In short, Foulkes conceptualized 'the mind of an individual person in terms of a personal matrix in the context of the collective mind of a grouping, characterised by a dynamic matrix in the context of a society, characterised by a foundation matrix' (ibid, p. 15). In the group situation, which Foulkes investigated through his invention of the T-situation (the group-analytic group), the three levels of the matrix can be seen as operating upon each other in recursive loops. Personal matrices feed into the dynamic matrix, which also feeds from the foundation matrix, and vice-versa. We will come back to the operational principles of the tripartite matrix in the context of the therapy zoo, later.

Let us first delve a little deeper into the foundation matrix. Here, Foulkes saw the pre-existing, relatively static, biological and cultural background of the individual, resonating 'down the generations' (ibid, p. 12) and transmitting the socio-cultural inheritance of the past into the here-and-now of the dynamic group matrix. The reference to both species elements and societal elements is somewhat blurred and confusing, and Foulkes has not given us much to work with. Understandably, most literature on the subject has focused on the socio-cultural aspect in humans, and neglected the species related biological and social aspects. Bacha (2019) makes an interesting connection between Foulkes's notions of the foundation matrix (Foulkes, 1973), his notion of the primordial level of communication (Power, 2017) and Panskepp's notion of the MindBrain (Panskepp, 2011). These concepts all refer to a socially and biologically inherited set of processes, involving emotional communication and patterns of interactions between embodied selves within a living community. 'Human and mammal emotions', she says, 'originate in distinguishable [neurological] pathways which are the same across individuals and across enormous swathes of time' (p. 6). This primordial level of both mental and neurological activity (hence: MindBrain, or BrainMind), which is essentially emotional and social, also cuts across species, with many resemblances, as well as differences, between individuals, communities and genomes. So, better informed than Foulkes was in his time, we can now therefore accept that any group of animals, merely being of the same class (e.g. *Mammalia*) or phylum (e.g. *Chordata*), share some basic fundamental mental matrix (foundational matrix).

What does this foundation matrix look like in a community of rabbits? Take a rabbit pen for example, with hutches, logs and straw bedding scattered around on the ground. In this wide, well protected and equipped pen lives a community of say 5–10 domesticated (pet) rabbits, bucks and does more or less evenly balanced. Much in common with their wild relatives, the Wild European Rabbits, they have a pecking order and a dominance hierarchy. The more dominant adults get to eat first, and the dominant male has mating rights with the females. The adult females show territorial behaviour around their hutches, especially during spring and summer, when they are busy lining their nests with hair pulled from their tummies. At such times, competitive and aggressive behaviours may erupt to establish dominance and mounting will appear as part of sexual or hierarchical transactions. In the presence of a perceived threat, rabbits thump the ground with their hind feet to communicate danger and scatter into their shelters. Play, care and grooming behaviours are also observable among rabbits in the community. In a cohesive pack with good living conditions, young rabbits race up and down and jump in the air, and older rabbits dig at the same hole, or rip up some old newspapers together. Rabbits groom each other as a sign of affection and generally spend a lot of time together, sleeping snuggled up against each other. This is the culture of the rabbit community, culture being here the biologically inherited social patterns and habits. All this is part of the foundation matrix in the rabbit pen and can be described in terms of a mental field, within which many interpersonal processes take place between individual minds grouped together, forming a dynamic network of ongoing communication.

How does the interplay between the three levels of the matrix occur in the rabbit community? Each rabbit has its own unique personality, influenced by its gender, age, breed, personal history and living conditions. On the mental level or the personal matrix, each rabbit perceives the social sphere via its internalised working models and reacts to social events by the activation of mental processes informed by implicit knowledge drawn from its own life experiences. Through its behaviour, the individual rabbit affects the dynamic matrix of the community at any given moment. If a human steps into the pen, for instance, the rabbits' reactions will vary between expressions of fear and curiosity, within the range dictated by their foundation matrix, depending on the norms and history of the specific community. Individual rabbits who feel safe around humans and anticipate positive feelings (potentially resulting from receiving physical or emotional nurturance) will bend the community norms towards approaching and gathering around the visitor, sniffing his hands, and seeking food and touch. Home-grown free-ranging rabbits are known for their tendency to include humans in their social hierarchy and to show positive attachment to humans, while rabbits who are raised alone in cages are known to show schizoid interpersonal styles and be more suspicious of both other rabbits and humans. Such individuals will affect the dynamic matrix of the pack in the direction of their personal perspectives, while at the same time driven to change their personal matrices according to the patterns of the group. Foulkes' basic law of group dynamics describes this interplay nicely: 'The deepest reason why [these] patients… can reinforce each other's normal reactions and wear down and correct each other's neurotic reactions, is that *collectively they constitute the very norm, from which, individually, they deviate*' (Foulkes, 1948, p. 29, my italics).

Communication in (e)motion

As shown in Chapter 4, the basic operating system of social organisms lies in the activation of emotional states in response to events in the external environment. Emotions are more ancient and are situated deeper in the brain than thoughts and cognitions. 'Emotions let us know that something is happening in our environments, in much the same way as pain or fever alert us to something happening in our bodies' (Bacha, 2019, p. 5). Emotions have a value tag attached to them, which tells us if what is happening is good or bad: whether to approach or to avoid. The foundational emotional systems are action-systems, activating 'intentions in action' (Panskepp, 2012). The basic emotions are thus expressed through the behaviour of the animal, transmitting its intention and appreciation of the situation. Those emotional behaviours become communicative actions as they are received by other organisms and take part in interpersonal/social interactions. The Latin origin of the word 'emotion' combines the prefix 'e', which means 'outwards', and the word 'movere' which is 'to move'. In French, the word is close to 'emouvir' which means to excite, or to stir-up. It underscores both the action and the interpersonal aspects of emotions. Emotions are therefore the fundamental currency in interpersonal communication among animals. They link the embodied nature of animal sociality, as described by Panskepp (ibid), with the mental field of communication (the matrix), described by Foulkes as operating in all groupings of minds (1973).

If the matrix is conceptualized as a transpersonal network of communication, then what flows through its channels, transmitted between and through its individual stations and intersections (or as Foulkes called it – the nodal points), is first and foremost the emotional states that arise in the social system at each specific point in place and time. Emotional states evoke thought patterns and mental activity that correspond to the emotional content and to the environmental circumstances in which it arose, within the limitations and inclinations of each individual from each species, and to the best of what its neurological apparatus can produce. While the working models and interpersonal patterns vary between any meeting of individuals, they all are part of the dynamic matrix and reflect the foundation matrix of the social system. In this context we speak of the emotional and mental state of a sub-group or the group-as-a-whole in any given moment. We see this clearly when we enter the rabbit pen with a bucket full of vegetables. The excitement that spreads throughout the pack is contagious, driving even the most timid of the rabbits to emerge from their hutches, stand up on their hind paws and sniff the air in curiosity. In this situation, we also will hardly remain indifferent and will most likely come to share the excitement that bubbles all around us. At times, only a part of the group will share a specific emotional state, while others will react differently or indifferently, such as when mating behaviours occur.

The therapy zoo is a grouping of a number of such communities. Some of them are confined to exclusive areas and some share a corral or an open space with other species. Open and shared areas serve as a 'market-place', with busy traffic and a variety of animals. This is the bedding in which the therapeutic dyad is conceived. The therapy sessions can be limited to specific niches or, as usually is the case, the child chooses the route and the rhythm of the session. And so the therapist accompanies the child in the early sessions, in his exploration of this new world into which he has landed. Many patients will spend their sessions hopping from one niche to another, visiting each habitat briefly and moving on, roaming the central scene, absorbing the culture and adjusting to the social atmosphere of the place. As they merge into the matrix, they develop their habits and create rituals. Their weekly visits become a routine. They get more and more involved and invested in interactions, adding to the matrix while being created by it, as does the therapist. The patient follows the therapist's lead in his first attempts to connect with animals, as the therapist follows the patient around. They are a pack of two. A pack with a dynamic matrix of its own. Gradually, the dyad finds itself spending more time in specific niches, to which they return at each session. The child now feels more at home in the therapy zoo, less like a newcomer and more like one of the locals. The relationship with the therapist deepens and her presence gives the child a sense of security that establishes his capacity to be alone (Winnicott, 1958), in the sense that he is freer to engage in emotional social interactions with the animals around him. His ability to explore his social surrounding in a playful, relatively anxiety-free state of mind depends on the mental maintenance of a transitional space, where he can begin working through the challenges that are re-enacted for him in his interactions with the animals he meets. In these interactions the patient experiences emotions and relives self-states of various kinds. His communicative gestures transmit those emotional states outwards. A flinch, a hesitating hand or a frozen posture while clinging to the therapist, as well as a carefree running around, chasing animals, distributing food or shoving hands inside a rabbit hatch, are all indicators that animals respond to with communicative gestures of their own. Emotions flow in the matrix, creating an emotional atmosphere that can be assessed by the therapist and discussed with the patient, improving her awareness of her own feelings and of the relational processes that take place around her. A myriad of relational events and emotional transactions present themselves to the child, with the assistance of the therapist, from which the child can choose the ones that carry the most relevance to the therapeutic goals.

The dyad-in-the-matrix

At this point, focusing on sequences of sessions in a certain community within the therapy zoo, we can speak of the nascence of a new clinical phenomenon, in which the therapeutic dyad becomes one with the animal community. Connections between humans and animals are now moulded into social patterns, enriching the dynamic matrix and affecting the personal matrices of individuals. Some animals may begin to show enthusiasm and greet the patient and/or therapist when they come on their weekly visit as if they were waiting for them, while others will learn to run and hide at the mere sight or sound of the child and/or adult approaching their niche. Sometimes the whole pack will experience a positive or negative transference towards the human dyad, and sometimes they will disregard them, treating them as inconsequential fellow animals that incidentally share the same space. The animals in the therapy zoo are accustomed to people engaging them to interact and may not at first distinguish one visitor from another. But as the session proceeds, this new social system, the dyad-in-the-matrix, will begin to exhibit its unique characteristics, some of which can be compared to the group-analytic model of the small analytic-group (the 'T-situation', Foulkes, 1986).

With regard to the treatment (T) situation, Foulkes devised a method in which a small group of strangers meets regularly and is encouraged to free-associate. He referred to the group therapist as a conductor, alluding to the conductor of an orchestra, once he realized that one of the therapist's missions is to intervene in ways that enhance the group's synchronicity, harmony and coherence (Foulkes, 1984; Pines, 1994). He says:

> With this orientation in the mind of the conductor, the group-analytic situation becomes the natural meeting ground of the biologist, anthropologist, sociologist and psycho-analyst. In fact, it displays the living process as what it really is – a co-ordinated and concerted whole (1984, p. 64).

One of the peculiar features of the group-analytic situation is its orientation towards a discussion which is 'completely loose and undisciplined, a free association of ideas, which can be best described as a "free-floating discussion"' (Foulkes, 1984, pp. 45–55). In the dyad-in-the-matrix group the dynamic field of interactions can be described in the same manner, although we are inclined to change the word 'ideas' to something less cognitive and more biologically oriented, like emotions or mental-states. In both situations the group is seen as a 'concerted whole' where each individual, human or animal, is looking to find its own way to fit in, thereby adding its 'colour', to the total picture. In the process of fitting in, the individual experiences a growing sense of coherence and a better understanding of what is going on (Pines, 1994). She becomes an active member, takes part in establishing the norms of the group and is corrected by the group when she deviates from these very norms (Foulkes, 1948). It is not just the conductor/therapist but the whole group, including the conductor/therapist, which is doing the therapeutic work. Each response by any participant to another constitutes an interpretation, mirroring or resonating with some aspect in the recipient (Foulkes, 1977), an aspect that the latter may not have been aware of, but which was communicated by his earlier gestures and processed and responded to by others.

The dyad-in-the-matrix within the animal community is very different from the analytic-group. While the group members in the analytic group are discouraged from, and even forbidden to communicate in any way other than through words and body language, in the new matrix that incorporates both human and animal, communication is not restricted to words, but encompasses all manners of interactions, including movement, touch and nonverbal voice-making. Interactions are hands-on, remain relatively simple most of the time and are based on emotional communication, given the paucity of wider foundational common grounds like language, culture and symbolic thinking. The dynamic matrix of the dyad-in-the-matrix is impregnated by forces belonging to the relational bio-social nature of all creatures in the matrix. It is nevertheless quite poor in the realm of words, symbols and ideas. This remains a private matrix of the therapeutic dyad, which holds the alpha function (Bion, 1967) in the transitional space, the place of birth and processing of ideas, the playground of the mind. Another difference is that the animals are not concerned with exploring their relations with each other and with the humans. They are action oriented and focus on the here and now only, monitoring a much narrower field. They usually don't care about and don't intentionally think of what they do or why they do it, whether in relation to humans or to other animals. The dyad, under the orchestration of the therapist, doesn't share with the animals the mental activity dedicated to the explorations of the social and psychological processes that touch the patient. It is not because they don't talk to the animals about it, but because the animals can't understand most of it.

Consequently, patients map the social climates of different niches and navigate the therapeutic dyad between them according to an inner campus. The patient chooses to visit specific individuals and/or groups who have captured their interest and who may be willing to engage with them socially, maintaining an ongoing relationship. It is important to remember that the clinical focus is still distinctly and unmistakably centred on the patient. In this model, the child patient is the one who experiences the maximal transformative effect of the group processes. Nevertheless, the animals and of course the therapist are also affected, and it is not uncommon that some animals, individuals and groups, benefit from the therapy with observable change.

Part II: Sara's journey: clinical illustration and discussion

The clinical material that will be presented below is based on extracts from the treatment of Sara in a therapy zoo. The details have been altered and personal features changed for confidentiality reasons. Following is a discussion of the material, using the theoretical perspective and terminology presented above.

Case study – Sara learns to play

Sara, 9 years old, is an only child with a mild developmental disorder. She was born with hypotonia and was late to reach all her developmental milestones. The challenges and hardships that her parents have gone through with Sara are the reason why they have decided not to bear more children. Sara has undergone all kinds of treatments and is reported to be cooperative because 'she understands that it's all for her own good'. At home, although quite able to do everything on her own, Sara is still assisted by her parents down to the minutiae of her daily chores (e.g., bathing, dressing and brushing her teeth). In school, she is struggling academically and participates in a special education program. Sara gets along socially but tends to be easily offended and seems meek and compliant with her peers. Generally, notwithstanding occasional bouts of distress, Sara is a happy girl without any signs of a major emotional disorder.

At the beginning of therapy, the therapist noticed that Sara loved feeding animals and showed no fear when they fought amongst themselves over the food. In fact, she found interesting ways to trigger these fights. She brought apples to the donkeys or collected carobs and hay for the goats and then went to the most crowded areas, where she distributed the food as evenly as she could. She then reprimanded the rude donkeys who took more for themselves at the expense of others and scolded the butting goats for their aggressiveness, ordering them to stop fighting. Sara was fascinated by the birds and it was as if an invisible force was drawing her again and again to the aviary. She liked standing in the middle of a flock of cockatiels holding a mixture of grains in her hand, choosing individual birds whom she had learned to identify by their colours and trying to feed them. This got the flock into a frantic dance of wing-flaps and screeches, creating around her a chaos of competition and pursuit. With a very serious face Sara talked to the cockatiel she was determined to feed and reached out to it with her palm full of grains. The frightened bird escaped, leaping from one branch to another, sometimes trying to bite her hand. Other cockatiels took shots at picking up grains from Sara's hand, which swung forth and back. The whole flock became aggressively ecstatic, while Sara remained cold and resolute and used her second hand to fend off the snatchers. She kept talking, addressed specific cockatiels or the group-as-a-whole, or talked partly to the therapist and partly to herself, as if narrating the choreography of the matrix in front of her.

> Please honey, you need to eat. Don't run away. Stop grabbing, you. It's not for you! You already got some, leave for the others. Look, they are fighting. This one is biting, be careful. Ah, you moved over here, now you want some? Here, come eat.

Similar scenes repeated themselves with the geese and ducks by the pond. The therapist intentionally stayed back most of the time, observing silently.

When a group of angry geese approached her once with menacing screeches and beak-strikes, Sara didn't pick-up on the threatening vibe and the therapist had to intervene. She pointed out to Sara that they are not asking for food but are actually communicating that they want her and the therapist to back off. But Sara wasn't available to notice that. She had to be gently removed to avoid herself being hurt.

Within a few weeks, it seemed that Sara was becoming aware of the emotional states in the animals around her and responded to them. Noticing their fear brought to the surface issues of competition and power. 'Who is the strongest?', 'who do you think?'. Sara named two donkeys, 'because they make the others scared.' 'Why are the others scared of them?' Sara couldn't say. On some occasions, when the goats broke into a fight, she asked to leave the scene, showing first signs of fear. She felt pity for Toby, a white male pygmy goat who was kept in seclusion and was thirsty for attention and she gave him weekly encouragements. In the chicken coop, there was a social structure that resembled a family, which led to a discussion on sibling rivalry and to Sara sharing that at home she has the TV all to herself with no one to fight her for it, 'except for when daddy wants it, and then I go to my parents' room, they also have a TV. It's more cosy there'. In the nursery, there were four chicks, two of them significantly bigger than the other two, who were newborns. She said the big ones are 'daddy and daddy' and was preoccupied by their size. Then she asked, 'why are they looking at me?'. She said they should have a slide so they can play. She then took the therapist to a slide in a corner of the therapy zoo, went up and sat down at the top. But she didn't slide down. She changed her mind and came down by the ladder. Then she headed to the pen to feed the goats. Passing by Toby, Sara said it must be that he is kept apart because he was being bullied, and now he is safe. Suddenly a group of peacocks came right through them. She had bread in her hand and began throwing pieces at them, saying 'take, take, just don't fight'. The blue ones, she explained, are the dads. 'My best friend A has no father. My father and I play ball together. Do you have a ball?' They then went to the playroom and got a ball and played passes until it was time to say goodbye. Sara's father then came in and she seemed to react with panic and embarrassment. Something that was released earlier was now restrained. She returned the ball to its place and went silently to join him.

One day she brought carobs to Toby, 'to make him happy'. The therapist asked, 'what else will make him happy?'. 'Company. If we play with him', Sara answered. After Toby had eaten, the therapist suggested they open the gate for him to walk around. Sara didn't resist. They followed Toby who took off in the direction of the pen where all the other goats were. Sara said he misses them, and that he is lonely. The therapist showed Sara how to caress and play with Toby by rubbing his forehead. They played together for a while and then resumed their stroll. Toby was now much calmer and more playful, exploring around himself but keeping a short distance away from Sara. After a while, Sara became anxious about him being out so long. She became bossy and started taking him back to his solitary enclosure. The therapist tried to appease her by saying that Toby could use the time-out after being closed in all day. Sara stopped and suddenly said that she also is alone a lot, when daddy is at work and mommy is cooking. She then relaxed and set Toby free, leaving him to visit other niches. In the next meeting, she went straight to Toby, who responded to the sight of Sara and the therapist approaching with loud excitation. She fed him and played with him. Watching them, the therapist thought that she had not seen Sara so playful and uninhibited previously. She let Toby nibble her shoelaces and stand up, laying his front paws on her chest. She answered in sweet words and caresses and rubbed his forehead. His affectionate attention filled her with joy. Then she let him out again and they strolled in the open area. It made her proud when she noticed that he was following her this time, and not the other way around, like last week.

Discussion

By choosing to bring such rich material my aim is to demonstrate the multi-layered therapeutic experience that the work in the therapy zoo can offer. I will not attempt to touch upon all that transpired in the vignettes that I have described. The following discussion will present the way that I think, as a clinician, while trying to make sense of what is going on, and to connect the personal and the interpersonal, and the matrix and the transitional space. My discussion also reflects a movement between languages and theoretical perspectives, integrating as it were the three axes of the theory of Animal-Assisted Therapy outlined in the previous and the present chapters.

The therapy zoo plays a leading role in Sara's therapy. It has a strong presence as an interactive environment (Roitman and Kassirer-Izraeli, 2013). It is characterized by responsivity and initiative, thus enhancing the relational aspect of the therapeutic process. As an analytic space, it is very much 'alive' and enlivens Sara's internal dramas, by facilitating the production of enactments with the participation of the animals. As a patient, Sara quickly let herself dive into a transitional space within the matrix and engaged in what relational analysts call 'play' (Frankel, 1998) with the animals. Disregarding social constraints, which demand some time and effort to remove in most children her age, Sara immediately went for contact with the animals in a way that conveyed the assertion that they are her equals. At first, she initiated interactions trying to control the situation by taking on the role of the giver. By possessing the goods, she made sure the others will be drawn to her. Still, she only managed to feel effective when she got the dynamic matrix intensely agitated. Her version of the giver role was a brilliant recapitulation of her mother, who hovered over her continuously to offer assistance. It also had some clear features of her father's authoritative manner. She didn't tolerate aggressiveness but kept inducing it, as part of the enactment that she created with the animals. The communities she frequented became enthusiastic in her presence. She could magically invoke a contagious SEEKING state (Panksepp, 2012) around her, spreading to all the participants but somehow not affecting her. Nor did she seem to be touched by the uneasiness that accompanied the aggressive side of the dynamic matrix that was being enacted. I believe this is a good example of a massive scale projective identification, or in the group-analytic nomenclature, a case of strong resonance in a group (Foulkes, 1977). We can ask how this kind of interaction affects the animal community's dynamic matrix over time, and how the personal matrices of the cockatiels, the geese, the donkeys, are changed by it. These questions are important as part of the ethical and zoological aspects of the therapist's work, but this is not the place to address them.

A few weeks into therapy Sara seemed to have descended one level deeper into the matrix. As a result, her awareness of others' feelings has opened, and her authoritative style has softened. She has mapped the therapeutic space and was now choosing a niche or specific animal to visit to match an internal state or need she experienced. She took the therapist with her in a journey through her internal zoo (Maayan, 2005), reflected on the encounters she had with animals in the real (external) zoo. It is clear that the therapist was now much more present as a subject for Sara, as were the animals. We can say that the dyad-in-the-matrix was now born. With the donkeys and the goats, a re-enactment of power struggles and anxieties related to oral-aggressive drives were featuring in the themes that resonated in the dynamic matrix. In Toby, Sara found mirroring for her socially rejected part, and in the chickens, a reflection of her longing for siblings, her fear of competition and her wish for father's attention. These projections, accompanied by behavioural gestures, were responded to by the animals, thereby co-creating relational moments in which Sara could explore and express her feelings and self-states, and work through some of her emotional and developmental challenges.

For example, when she talked about giving the chicks a slide to play, she was probably referring to her own wish and difficulty in playing, which was connected in her mind to the longing for siblings and to her ambivalence towards her father, who represented for her alternatively a daunting authority and a play partner. In my mind, this is the context of her change of heart on the top of the slide. Sara is a girl who can't play as freely as other children do. We know that the emotional state of PLAY (Panskepp, 2012) requires a specific relational context in which to evolve into the socially expected capacity to play. The context of the therapy zoo can encourage children to develop this capacity, by giving them both the incentive and the relational context they require. Note the interplay between the effects of the animals on Sara and her ability to make use of the therapist as a developmental agent. I am addressing here the observable fact that Sara's invitation to the therapist to play ball, maybe the first time she had done this since the beginning of therapy, was preceded by the feelings that were aroused in her while watching and interacting with the 'family' of chickens. Here, Sara's personal matrix fed into the dynamic matrix, also fed by the foundation matrix of the chickens, and a re-enactment of a scene from Sara's relationship with her father emerged. It also demonstrates a sequence beginning in the interpersonal, touching the personal and resounding back to the interpersonal. This back and forth resonance of emotional interplay of self-states, or object-relational patterns, occurs in the transitional space inside Sara's mind and in the context of a set of communicational processes occurring in the matrix. What was exchanged here were emotional states, which regulated the emotional state of the group, or sub-groups, by activating PLAY states and soothing FEAR states. Sara's reaction to her father stepping in shows a reverse effect.

Pulling just one more of many possible threads, I want to focus on another sequence, involving Sara, Toby and the therapist. In the first session of the two reported, Sara decides to go and make Toby happy by feeding him. The therapist, holding in mind her social difficulties and her sensitivity to Toby's need for company and attention, interprets in the form of a leading question, 'what else will make him happy?'. Sara immediately understands, and by that acknowledges the containment of her own similar need by the therapist. She goes on feeding Toby, still treating his loneliness, but unable to connect to her own vulnerability. The therapist then intervenes again, opening a concrete as well as a metaphoric gate. And then, another intervention is needed on her part, in order to show Sara a way to engage Toby in play. Her interventions affect both Toby and Sara, building a bridge connecting both their needs to interact more intimately with each other. She models for Sara how to play with Toby, thereby impacting the dynamic matrix towards increased degrees of freedom, playfulness and intimacy. Sara is finally able to relinquish the safe position of 'giver' and meet Toby from a more equal and vulnerable position. Toby also gives up his plan to join the other goats, turning instead to Sara whom he now sees as a playmate. Their play is therapeutic for both, but Sara still can't hold it for long. While Toby seems to have relaxed and is joyfully prancing around, Sara resumes her adult-like manner and soon becomes anxious, as if she did something wrong and is about to get castigated. A surge of guilt and anxiety drives Sara to take Toby back and lock him up. I believe that this was a transformative moment, beginning with a possibly malignant form of projective identification between Sara and Toby, but which was then resolved by the therapist, in her statement that Toby would actually prefer staying out than being locked up again. By giving words to Toby's subjectivity, she helped Sara regain empathic connection with herself and an implicit memory surfaced, that of Sara's feelings of loneliness in her own home. In the next session, Sara and Toby are anxious to meet again and repeat the pleasurable experience of playing together. Their personal matrices have incorporated something from the dynamics of the last session and are feeding into the dynamic matrix of the here-and-now. For Sara, it was a revelation to realise that she is wanted and loved by her peers and that she can be a leader, not just a follower, in her relationships with them.

Part III Summary

Thinking within the framework of the dyad-in-the-matrix enables us to encompass and analyse various processes, both intra-psychic and interpersonal, that take place simultaneously in a child-therapy in a therapy zoo. I have found that although such processes as those depicted in the above case study are common in AAP, we have so far been short of an appropriate theoretical framework and terminology to address them. Especially with regard to the relational and social processes in which the animals are taking an important part. It is my impression that today, still, every AAP therapist and supervisor must invent his or her own nomenclature to think about and discuss analytically what is going on in therapy, beyond the merely behavioural concepts of causality and conditioning.

The suggested approach can be applied to group therapy in a therapy zoo, as well as to individual therapy involving a single animal, say when a dog takes part in the psychotherapy of a child in a playroom, or outdoors. In any case, it may be useful to begin by assessing and mapping the various matrices that are present, and the interplay between them. As far as the technical implications that this has on the work of the clinician, these may affect mostly the way we think and to what we attend to. I believe that most experienced AAP therapists working in therapy zoos have developed strong intuitions as to how to intervene in ways that facilitate and enhance the therapeutic process. This has to do with the fact that they have themselves become part of the matrix of their working environment, affecting and being affected by it. This has inevitably impacted their personal matrices in ways that help them 'read' in richer and more sophisticated ways the human-animal multifaceted matrix in which each dyad-in-the-matrix is conceived, born and developed throughout the therapy. What we need most urgently now is a comprehensive theory to explain how it all works and provide us with the words to communicate it.

The therapeutic journey of Noah's Ark concludes with the arc-in-the-sky covenant, where God says: *(9)*[12] ... *This is the token of the covenant which I make between me and you and every living creature that is with you, for perpetual generations:*[13] *I do set my bow in the cloud, and it shall be for a token of a covenant between me and the earth.*

Here, we are reminded of the larger context, uniting all living things under God's eyes. The story of Noah's Ark therefore marks an awakening of the awareness of the foundation matrix connecting the whole animal kingdom, to which mankind also belongs.

Notes

1 Parallel myths from other cultures, such as the Mesopotamian, the Greek and the Persian, are slightly different but preserve most basic motives of the story. Interestingly, all avoid going into the details of what the passengers of the ark went through during the deluge and the great flood.
2 In awareness of the on-going debate about gender issues, references to the patient and the therapist, when a gender isn't specified, will be either in male or female terms. They should be read as referring to both genders.

References

Bion, W. R. (1967) *Second thoughts*. London: Heinemann.

Brown, D. (1994) Self-development through subjective interaction: A fresh look at ego training in action. In: D. Brown and L. Zinkin (Eds.), *The psyche and the social world: Developments in group-analytic theory*. London: Routledge, pp. 80–98.

Foulkes, S.H. (1948) *Introduction to group-analytic psychotherapy: Studies in the social integration of individuals and groups*. London: Maresfield Reprints.

Foulkes, S.H. (1973) The group as matrix of the individual's mental life. In: L. R. Wolberg and E. K. Schwartz (Eds.), *Group therapy: An overview*. New York: Intercontinental Medical Book Corporation. pp. 223–233.

Foulkes, S.H. (1977) Notes on the concept of resonance. In: L.R. Wolberg and M. L. Aronson (Eds.), *Group therapy 1977: An overview*. New York: Stratton Intercontinental, pp. 52–58.

Foulkes, S.H. (1984) *Therapeutic group analysis*. London: Karnac.

Foulkes, S.H. (1986) *Group analytic psychotherapy: Method and principles*. London: Routledge.

Frankel, J.B. (1998) The play's the thing. How the essential processes of therapy are seen most clearly in child therapy. *Psychoanalytic Dialogues*, 8(1), pp. 149–182.

Fuchs, S.H. (1938). ber Den Prozess Der Zivilisation 1st Vol.: Wandlungen Des Verhaltens in Den Weltlichen Oberschichten Des Abendlandes: By Norbert Elias (Academia Verlag Prag Vorabdruk, 1937, pp. 327). *International Journal of Psycho-Analysis*, 19, pp. 263–265.

Hopper, E. (2018) The development of the concept of the tripartite matrix: A response to 'Four modalities of the experience of others in groups' by Victor Schermer. *Group Analysis*, 51(2), pp. 197–206.

Lavie, J. (2005) The lost roots of the theory of group analysis: Taking interrelational individuals seriously! *Group Analysis*, 38(4), pp. 519–535.

Maayan, E. (2005) Inside and outside in animal-assisted therapy: The inner reality meets the external reality of the therapy zoo. *Haiot Vehevra (Animals and Society)*, 27(1), pp. 57–66 [In Hebrew].

Mead, G.H. (1934) *Mind, self and society*. Chicago, IL: University of Chicago Press.

Nitzgen, D. and Hopper, E. (2018) The concepts of the social unconscious and of the matrix in the work of S. H. Foulkes. In: *The social unconscious in persons, groups and Societies: Volume 3: The foundation matrix extended and re-configured*. New York: Routledge, pp. 3–26.

Panksepp, J. (2011) Cross-species affective neuroscience decoding of the primal affective experiences of humans and related animals. *PLoS One*, 6(9), e21236. doi:10.1371/journal.pone.0021236.

Panksepp, J. (2012) A synopsis of affective neuroscience: Naturalizing the mammalian brain. In "The philosophical implications of affective neuroscience." *Journal of Consciousness Studies*, 19(3–4), pp. 6–18.

Pines, M. (1994) The group-as-a-whole. In: D. Brown and L. Zinkin (Eds.), *The psyche and the social world: Developments in group-analytic theory*. London: Routledge, pp. 48–60.

Power, K. (2017) On the primordial origins of group analysis and their relation to the creative nature of humanity. *Group Analysis*, 50(1), pp. 91–103.

Roitman, D. and Kassirer-Izraeli, H. (2013) The therapeutic setting as a living presence: Considerations on child psychotherapy in a therapy zoo. *Sihot (Conversations)*, 28(1), pp. 67–76 [In Hebrew].

Stacey, R. (2001) What can it mean to say that the individual is social through and through? *Group Analysis*, 34(4), pp. 457–471.

Winnicot, D.H. (1958) The capacity to be alone. *International Journal of Psycho-Analysis*, 39(4), pp. 416–420.

7 Unexpected objects in the group

The Foulksian group-analytic boundary

David Vincent

This chapter considers a problem for group psychotherapists: where does the group begin and end? What is inside the group, and what is outside? What is it that separates inside and outside and keeps them apart, as you cannot see or touch the boundary? There are various ways of thinking about this: is it a membrane, as in a cell, or is it a skin, like a body? Is it a fence, a border or a boundary? Or is it simply a conscious understanding between the members of the group, as in a gang or a club? All humans have a natural tendency to join together in small groups and to immediately have a sense of the group as a whole and its difference and separation from, and possibly rivalry with, other groups. In other words, the group immediately knows its boundary. This applies to all human groups, and to all psychotherapy groups.

This chapter is about three 'boundary incidents', unexpected intrusions into the group by animals: a hornet, some baby budgies and a companion dog. In each case, the intrusion became both a kind of 'enactment' and an experience of triangulation, a kind of thirdness, and resulted in emotional, relational progress in the group, a growth in understanding both for the individual patients and for the group as a whole. There are very few references to group psychotherapy in relational theory compared to the richness of individual relational theory, and yet what could be more relational than a group? The analyst or therapist in a group in fact has little choice. In front of them, relational dilemmas are continually enacted between and by the members of the group. I have argued elsewhere that triangulation (thirdness) is a building-block of the group, which continually develops from two-person to three-person relationships and back again (Vincent, 2016).

Group analysis

S. H. Foulkes, the founder of Group Analysis, was a psychiatrist and a psychoanalyst. He thought that the 'free-floating conversation' in the group was the exact equivalent of 'free association' in individual psychoanalysis. Freud's 'fundamental rule' (Freud, 1912, p. 107) and the connected basis of technique, 'evenly suspended at attention' (Freud, 1912), therefore, for Foulkes, could also both apply in group analytic psychotherapy.

In psychodynamic, psychoanalytic or group-analytic group psychotherapy, the distinguishing feature of the work, compared to all other kinds of group therapy, is the emphasis on the unconscious. The aim and drive of the therapeutic work are to get to know and understand both individual and group unconscious wishes, thoughts and fantasies. As in individual psychoanalytic psychotherapy, the major part of this work lies in the consideration of childhood, sexuality, family relationships, dreams, fantasies and daydreams. These can then be brought into the present moment through the transference, both to the group psychotherapist and to the group. The work of the psychotherapist is to see and consider this in the light of their countertransference, their reverie and their analytic internal working model. In group psychotherapy, the psychotherapist is also pushed along by the continuous lively re-enactment in front of them, in the group, of family and other relationships. An individual patient talking about their jealousy, for example, of a sibling is painful to hear, but in group psychotherapy, this jealousy and the accompanying hatred and aggression are alive, at the moment, acted out in the room. Group psychotherapists will know that a new member of the group will always excite, for example, in the group the loving interest, envious curiosity and jealous hostility that meets a new baby in the family.

How does the psychotherapist enable this access to the unconscious life of the patient in the individual session or in the group? The first two factors are the psychotherapist's curiosity and their internal working model and the third factor is the psychotherapist's robustness. This is sorely tested in a group. It is difficult enough when an individual patient, for instance, strongly resists an interpretation, but if a whole group together, angrily or complacently, refuse to accept the view of the group psychotherapist, it can be hard to keep on track. Bion describes this feeling when he says that he felt that he had 'committed blasphemy in a group of true believers' and in the same paper, he advises the psychotherapist to 'throw off the numbing feeling of reality' (Bion, 1961, pp. 148–149). This is useful advice. It is precisely at those moments in the group when the group-as-a-whole confidently assert their view that they are right, that the psychotherapist must work hard to remember who and where they are. This is not a normal interaction, or 'the real world', and the group are fiercely resisting knowing something about themselves both as individuals and as a group, for fear of the anxiety that knowledge may provoke.

If the psychotherapist is curious, confident in their understanding of unconscious processes and robust enough, then what else is important? After these qualities of the psychotherapist, the next important matter is what is usually called the 'setting'. In group psychotherapy, this includes the 'boundary'. This, like the other necessary factors, facilitates, allows and encourages the expression and consideration of unconscious processes and the internal world of the patient. The most obvious factors of the setting are, as in all psychotherapy, neutrality, safety, quiet, confidentiality and regularity.

As far as possible, the setting is always the same. In group psychotherapy, this may be more difficult to achieve. Group members may be early or late, they may meet one another outside the group or on the way in and they may each, individually, have a reason for disrupting the group at some point, by being late, by rushing out in a rage, bringing in food or drink, picking a fight or arriving drunk or drugged. The group-as-a-whole can also disrupt the setting as part of a concerted campaign against the group psychotherapist by all arguing, for example, that it is perfectly normal to have biscuits and hot drinks in the group and offer to bring them in themselves next week. Part of their argument is often that this will help the work of the group, that it is normal, part of the 'real world', and that the group psychotherapist should therefore agree, and be grateful for their advice. At any point in the group, of course, if this argument seems to be convincing to the psycho-therapist, then they must immediately call Bion to mind, and 'throw off the numbing feeling of reality' (1961).

The setting includes the physical arrangements in the group room. This can very concretely embody the boundary, frame and body of the group, as the couch over time, in individual psychotherapy, comes to represent the mother's and analyst's body. As in an individual consulting room, the walls of the group room provide protection from the outside world, both real and imagined. They embody confidentiality and safety over time, and the sepa-rateness and uniqueness of this group, compared to all the others. The door of the group room therefore becomes invested with unusual importance as the portal to the other or 'real' world outside the group.

An established group learns to mutually protect the whole group setting by arriving on time and not leaving until the end. Group members often describe their apprehension in approaching the group room door when late, dreading the way the group would all turn to look as they entered. For group members who are often late, this may be what they are unconsciously creat-ing for themselves through their lateness. One patient, who was always late for the group, described how frightening this was when all the heads turned towards him as he came in, but it was at the same time a confirmation of his very depressed conviction that no one ever thought about him unless he was not there.

The group room also contains a circle of chairs, a small table in the mid-dle and perhaps some pictures on the wall. Hopefully, there is a window or a skylight to remind the group that there is also a world outside. But, if over time, the room begins to become increasingly useful to the group as a vehicle for both individual and group-as-a-whole projections, then some-times the outside world, even if only briefly glimpsed through a window, can be changed to suit the emotional life of the group or the individual at that moment.

One group took place in a room overlooking a small courtyard in a hos-pital. A member of the group noticed that two people were in the courtyard, talking to one another and apparently examining the plants in the flowerbed.

The group stopped talking and all turned to look out of the window at the unexpected visitors. The two visitors were oblivious to this interest and after a few moments walked away around the corner of the building. I assumed that they were two long-stay patients from the main hospital and I looked back at the group to find that their mood had changed. They began to talk to one another, in a thoughtful, reflective, musing way, on what had just happened and what they had seen. It gradually emerged that they had all seen different things: two men, two women, a couple, old and young people, patients, nurses and visitors. No one ever came to the courtyard again in the life of this group, but this odd exchange deepened the reflective capacity of this group so that they could better understand that what they saw was always partly what they wanted or needed to see, and that this could also apply to the group here in the room, as well as the world outside.

The exoskeleton

This is an example of what started as a rather ordinary intrusion into the on-going life of the group but which went on to have an important effect on one patient and the group's relationship with him. This group session took place in a large room in the old hospital building during the summer. The room had large glass doors, which looked out on a wild garden, full of wildlife. Foxes would often run by the doors, and the garden was full of birds.

One morning a very large hornet appeared in the group. It flew noisily around the room as we talked. Each time that someone spoke, the hornet seemed to fly towards their face, as though attracted by the sound. Gradually the group gave up and sat in silence staring at the hornet. They were amused to watch it fly at my face each time when I tried to make a comment. I thought, rather anxiously that I should do something about the hornet's intrusion, as it fell under what the group analysts call 'dynamic administration' (Foulkes, 1990, p. 173). I should not let the hornet spoil the group. The door of the room opened onto a busy corridor, and if I opened the door to shoo it out I would be compromising the boundary of the group, inviting the people in the corridor to look in and intrude. The windows were rusted and therefore kept shut. I decided that my only choice was to swat the hornet and take the consequences. I stood up and took up a newspaper that was lying on a chair. The group were silent and staring intently at me as I waited for the hornet to come in range, and then I swatted at it with the newspaper. Each time that I missed, the group stared at me more intently. Finally, I managed to knock the hornet down at the side of the room, where there was wooden flooring and no carpet. I saw that the hornet was still alive, struggling on the floor. I thought for a moment and then decided to step on it. Because of its size and the hollow wooden floor, there was a very loud crunching sound. An appalled silence followed, and no one moved. After a moment a patient said, very loudly: 'Aahh! The crunch of an exoskeleton!'

After a thoughtful pause, the group began to talk, rather to my surprise, as I was expecting the group to freeze and to cast me in the role of a cruel, murderous assassin, extinguishing individual life in pursuit of the perfection of the group, and I said this, only for it to be ignored. The group, as is often the case, were interested in their own work, and not in me. To them, I had just done my job as the group therapist and let them get on with it. The patient, Simon, who had made the remark about the exoskeleton was particularly lively and relaxed. He was an intelligent and complex man, in middle age, then about halfway through his four years in the group. He had a difficult early life. He was born just after the war, during which his parents had lost their first two young children, a baby and a toddler, when their house was bombed, and a wall fell over onto the children's bedroom, killing them. As he grew up he was continually compared unfavourably to the dead children, particularly to the toddler, whose photographs were everywhere in the family home. This never abated, and he recalled to the group that when he was bullied at school, as at home by his mother, he could never fight back and always gave in, protected only by a persistent fantasy that Superman would fly down and rescue him. He had a successful professional life as a technician but was not able to sustain personal relationships, mainly because of his persistent feeling that he could never be as good as his dead brother.

Shortly before the hornet incident, Simon had told the group about a vividly remembered incident from his childhood. He was about seven years old and in the course of building work at home, a large pile of sand had been left in the garden. He took his sea-side bucket and spade, and his teddy-bear, out into the garden and started to play with the sand, burying the teddy and digging him up again. His mother saw him from the kitchen window and ran out into the garden, shouted angrily at Simon, and seized the bucket, spade and teddy bear and threw them into the coal-fire. The group were moved by this story and began to relate to Simon more closely. They understood that Simon was unconsciously repeating and repairing the traumatic loss of the two babies, crushed under the bombed wall, by burying and digging up the teddy bear in the pile of sand, and that this was unbearable for his mother. A few weeks later Simon started to talk for the first time about his father, now dead, who was distant, but caring, also traumatised by the early loss of the children, but not inclined to continually upbraid Simon. He had managed to hold onto one connection with his father, a single button from his Merchant Navy uniform, and as he talked, he brought it out of his pocket to show us. Again, the group were touched by his trust in them, and he by their interest in him. The hornet incident occurred soon after this, and it is clear that what he was telling us then, was that his own exoskeletal character-formation, his 'character armour' (Reich, 1945), was starting to break down and give way in the group, where he was seen, perhaps for the first time, just for himself. On his last day in the group he told us that he had recently appeared in the audience on a television programme about psychotherapy. When the group asked him if he wasn't afraid to be recognised, he explained that he had deliberately worn a very brightly coloured shirt. He thought that the shirt might distract viewers from actually looking at him. The group were not convinced by this, it seemed to be a regression to his split view of himself, and they asked him then if he felt better for being in the group for four years. "Oh, yes," he said "Very much better. I have really changed, but not in any of the ways that I thought I would change".

This was important for the group to hear. A major part of being open to change in psychotherapy is being open to the thought that the original idea of change has itself to be changed. It may be a basic relational idea that the aim of therapy is continually intersubjectively renegotiated. This patient was finally able to do this and to let go of some of the phantasies of being able to put right the family trauma by splitting himself and pretending to be a character that he was not. The extent of the trauma gave rise to the extent of the character rigidity that was itself deforming and counter-productive. His movement through this process was helped in the middle stages of his group therapy by the incident with the hornet, in which he was able to say out loud and thereby confirm that he was beginning to relinquish his own exoskeleton, and that it sounded good (the "crunch"). The hornet, in this sense, represented a kind of 'thirdness' in the group. This momentarily freed both Simon and the group, who could then hear it as a confirmation of their work together. The group also perhaps had its own exoskeleton, an unconsciously intersubjectively assumed kind of brittle relating, which they could relinquish. They could then forgive my cruelty to the hornet, or, in other words, the group.

Addiction to regret

This second example of a helpful breach of the boundary also concerns a difficult, complex patient in a long-term group. The patient was an eccentric clever woman in the middle age. She was the only child of elderly socially awkward parents, now both dead. The patient, Jennifer, lived on her own and had never had a relationship. She had been referred to with long-term depression and social inhibition and was very apprehensive about joining a group. At first, she was stiff and uncommunicative, and only occasionally whispered a few words. Fortunately, most of the other group members were, in various ways, as troubled as her, and they were pleasant to her, and encouraging when she did speak, but really they just got on with their group, to which they were, at this time, very attached. Too much fuss, at the start of the group, would have undoubtedly put Jennifer off, and so for several months she just watched and listened and occasionally mumbled a comment. Somehow this was just what she needed, and she clearly felt gradually drawn into the unique and complex life of the group. She had a range of health problems for which she consulted with doctors, but didn't receive diagnoses or treatment. She then began to speak about this, finding her first real spoken involvement in the group in a vigorously shared series of complaints about the inadequacy of medical services. Almost all of the other group members had health problems, usually a mixture of diagnosable illness, psychosomatic complaints and depression. This allowed the group to show a lively interest in her, to engage her and to recruit her to their stringent views about the inadequacy of doctors, and, of course, psychotherapists.

She began to emerge, and in one group spoke at some length about her leg. She often looked uncomfortable and seemed to limp slightly. She explained that she had had a painful leg for a long time, after helping to push-start a car, which she could subsequently not fully bend for fear of pain, and for which she could get no help. Finally, a few years before joining the group, someone, perhaps a doctor, had advised her to have a very hot bath and to stretch out the leg in the bath. This had been a disastrous suggestion, and the leg had, by her account, painfully seized up for good. The group enjoyed this story and rallied around her. This had two consequences: the first was that she was finally able to ask us if she could put her leg up in the group on a stool, to which we agreed, and second, that it revealed an important part of her psychological life, with which the group identified, and which become a part of this group's unique language, that we called 'addiction to regret'. In this first account of her leg, she bitterly complained: 'If only I had not straightened my leg...' and this frequent repetition of 'if only I had not done this or that...' became a theme for her and the group, a kind of repetitive magical defence against the demands of reality.

Asking for the stool on which to put her leg, so that it could become obviously present in every group, was very important, as it allowed her to make a claim for attention which she was as yet unable to do by talking. None of the stools in the clinic seemed adequate to the task, so the next week she brought a square plastic bucket from home, which, inverted in front of her chair, was perfect. This then gave rise to the next problem: where could she keep the bucket as it was too awkward for her to take it home every week on the bus? I suggested that she consult the clinic domestic, a kind and thoughtful woman, who subsequently found Jennifer an empty cupboard off the waiting room, which was perfect. The group were pleased, something important had happened, a complex anxiety had been concretely contained (the bucket in the cupboard), Jennifer felt she had a place in the clinic, and we could move on.

Gradually, the group began to sense that there was an undescribed difficulty in Jennifer's early life, concerned with her father and that this connected with her leg, as it was her father's car that she had tried to push. The group began to see how angry she was and how difficult it was for her to show it. A new patient then joined the group, a very loud, choleric man with a severe obsessional neurosis. By this time, we knew a little more about Jennifer, and she was, in turn, very involved in the lives of the other members of the group. Outside of the group animals were more available to her affectionate interest. She first told us about her love for foxes, and how she left food out for them in the neighbourhood and worried about their illnesses. She also revealed to us that she was extremely interested in budgerigars and had been for some years trying to breed a perfectly blue budgie. The group enjoyed this, it seemed hopeful, generative and reparative. Having talked for a couple of sessions about a new clutch, about which she was very optimistic, one day, very excited, she brought the baby budgies to the group in a little cage to show us. We admired them and she put the cage on a chair at the side of the room. The group started and very quickly our new member, the obsessional man, fell into a rage about something that he was telling us and started shouting loudly. The budgies woke up, alarmed, and squawked. Jennifer, enraged on behalf of her budgies, sat up, pointed at the obsessional man and, at the top of her voice, shouted: 'Now look what you've done!' Silence fell, the obsessional man looked abashed, and the group stared in admiration at Jennifer.

After this incident, in which Jennifer contacted her rage for the first time in the group, enabled by the thirdness of the budgies, our relationship with her changed. She began to seem generally more real and more reachable. We never really understood her leg and what it symbolised, but the group now allowed this to be explored a little. Previously, if I had attempted to look for the unconscious meaning of the stiff leg, for example by trying to link the leg with a fantasy about her father's penis, then the group would vigorously interrupt: 'there you go again...where did you get that idea from...you are spoiling the mood'. The group would together protect Jennifer, whom they saw as fragile, by keeping me in check. It is always interesting when this happens in a long-term group as the group may see something about a group member that the group analyst has missed. After this boundary incident, the group seemed to feel that it was no longer necessary to protect Jennifer so much after they had seen her in a rage, and they therefore were less inclined to obstruct me on her behalf. With further assistance from both Jennifer and the irritable obsessional man, the group moved on.

The helpful dog

In a different group was a woman patient, Mary, disabled by childhood polio. She came to the group in a motorised wheelchair with a companion dog. The dog was mature, serious and self-composed. His job was to be a useful companion, to open doors and pick up objects, and generally to keep an eye on his owner. This group contained troubled, vulnerable people, and they were, as a consequence, conservative in their group behaviour, sitting, for example, in the same chairs each week. One man, Len, always sat in the corner of the room. He was rather paranoid in character and employed both reticence and elaborate intellectual defences to keep the group at a distance. He in particular said very little about his immediate family. The group did know that a few months before this group his mother had been unwell.

At the start of each group, the dog would walk slowly around the room glancing at each group member in turn. He would then lie down next to Mary's wheelchair for the duration of the group, only glancing up at her every now and again to check on her. If she became distressed then he would sit up and stare at her very intently until she recovered, and then he would lay down again. On this occasion when the group were assembled, he did his normal slow circular inspection. When he had gone around he turned back, and, instead of joining his owner, he went and lay down next to Len's chair, and then did not move. The group fell silent and stared at the dog and at Len. After a few moments, the group began to talk and wondered what this meant. Len was anxious and disconcerted. The group pressed him to say what was happening, and after some pressure, finally, reluctantly and awkwardly, he told us that his mother had just died. He was not going to speak of it, he said, his feelings were too strong, but the dog lying down next to him had been a shock. The group became moved by Len's plight, his inability to show feelings and his successful suppression of this sudden grief, which the group and I had missed completely. Only the dog knew that something was wrong and offered his close attention to Len. This was the only occasion, in two years of attendance, that the dog sat anywhere but next to his owner. The group were profoundly moved by the dog's sensitivity to Len's suffering. It showed them what can be hidden from and missed by the group. The group perhaps learned more from this than Len, who was still mostly hidden. He became a little more communicative, although rarely spontaneous. The group, however, began to be more sensitive both to the mood in the room and to the unspoken feelings.

The boundary of the group: conclusions

These three very ordinary incidents, when 'unexpected objects' appeared in long-term psychotherapy groups, show the importance of the group's boundary. In these examples, the breach of the boundary was by an insect, some birds and a dog. These three creatures kept it simple. If it is true that 'the group – and not the group therapist – is the agent of personal change' (Ormont, 2001, p. 38), then the establishment and protection of the boundary and the understanding of the unexpected intrusions are of central importance. The world of a small group is overwhelmingly a relational world; it contains and displays at the same time the internal social worlds of each individual member of the group, the continuous life of the social world outside and around the group, and lived in the moment in the group, the recreated, re-experienced interpersonal life of the past.

The significance of the boundary for situations such as these is marked by the use of the term 'boundary incident' by group analysts to describe the breach of a boundary. In the three incidents described here, the fact of a very small and harmless breach, by an alive but non-human object, confirmed for both the group-as-a-whole and the individuals involved, including the psychotherapist, both the strength and the importance of the boundary, and had a marked effect on the subsequent feeling-life of the group.

References

Bion, W.R. (1961) *Experiences in Groups.* London: Tavistock.

Foulkes, E. (ed.) (1990) *Selected Papers of S.H. Foulkes: Psychoanalysis and Group Analysis.* London: Karnac.

Freud, S. (1912) in *Complete Works, SE*, Vol. 12. London: Vintage.

Ormont, L. (2001) *The Technique of Group Treatment.* Madison, WIS: Psychosocial Press.

Reich, W. (1945) *Character Analysis.* New York: Simon and Schuster.

Vincent, D. (2016) Couple and Family Dynamics and Triangular Space in Group Psychotherapy. In Novakovic, A. (ed.), *Couple Dynamics.* London: Karnac, pp. 125–143.

8 Trauma inevitably equates to baggage[1]

Jo Frasca

Of the prolific criteria for a diagnosis of chronic post-traumatic stress disorder (PTSD), regrettably, she met most. The diagnosis was determined, using the internationally recognised reference in mental health, The Diagnostic and Statistical Manual of Mental Disorders III (1994).

In training, we were encouraged to think beyond the rigorous parameters of the DSM. While diagnosis is important and a useful tool, it is not always definitive. 'A patient is more than a series of diagnoses and words', our trainers would remind us. To keep the formal diagnosis in context we were encouraged to do our DSM reading and study in not-so elaborate a place such as a toilet, thereby limiting its overrated esteem. My trainers' caution has proved to be prudent. I use the past tense to refer to the DSM which, while still used by many, due to its controversial content has fortunately lost much of its power, control and the stronghold bestowed on it by the mental health profession. The currency of this document is now being plagued with contention around who might be driving the text's extensive diagnoses and disorder lists in order to profit financially (Greenberg, 2010, 2013; Reese, 2013; Frances, 2013). It is the preferred tool in the United States on account of its affiliation with psychiatry, mental health, and the insurance and pharmaceutical companies, though its predominance here is also wavering (ibid). It is not my intention to explore the controversy and arguments in this chapter, but only to note that there is a shift away from the use of the DSM as an exclusive diagnostic tool.

Referring in this case, however, to that very DSM, the following features described her behaviour: 'Experienced, witnessed, or was confronted with an event or events that involved actual or threatened death or serious injury, or a threat to the physical integrity of self or others' (DSM-III, 1994, p. 427). Many of her symptoms extended beyond those required to meet the diagnosis of PTSD. I noted with apprehension that she also suffered acute hypervigilance, an exaggerated startle response which I later learnt was caused by people smashing up her family home, and an avoidance of certain people, places and things, especially where there appears to be a re-enactment of a threat, or possible threat, aggression and/or violence. She constantly cowered when faced with unfamiliar locations and people, and she would flee the scene at the slightest sound.

This was the introduction to my new, incidental canine companion, Saydee.

When Saydee began realising that my home was her new home and that I was now her human mother, she appeared to find it distressing to have me out of her sight and she tended to become upset and agitated if I was not in her direct line of view. It was disheartening to see that in the list of symptoms she also met a diagnosis of separation anxiety. Freud considered babies as having instinctual impulses, where 'something inherent, wired in, prestructured, is pushing from within' (in Mitchell, 1988, p. 3). Mind for Freud emerges in the form of 'endogenous pressures' (ibid), that contribute to the trauma when the baby is left alone, while Bowlby (1973), and ultimately Mitchell (1988) suggest that the infant's habit of seeking proximity to the main carer is 'fundamentally dyadic and interactive' and that 'above all else [it] seeks contact ... and ... engagement with other minds' (1988, p. 3).

Bowlby (1973) explains that when the child is separated for longer than tolerable periods or finds themselves in unfamiliar and uncomfortable environments without the mother, they become anxious. If this period is brief the child can recover, re-attach and avoid a lifetime of emotional detachment. However, if the reverse occurs and the mother is unavailable for longer periods the child passes through three developmental phases: protesting the missing mother; despairing she will ever return, and finally, becoming detached. If the mother's absence becomes a pattern for the child, the child develops a more acute anxiety, often developing the symptoms in line with separation anxiety (ibid). Such was the case with Saydee. Saydee would pace and fret even if a short distance separated us and even if I was still in full view. She did not like being left anywhere, except with the people who had originally rescued her. Saydee was also a bed-wetter, although the people who rescued her told me she had only wet in fear. In our home, this also occurs when I am gone for longer than tolerable periods. It has not been a difficult task to overlay Saydee's anxious and distressed behaviours onto the developmental stages of children where separation creates many and varied symptoms, such as anxiety, bed-wetting, nightmares, cowering and acting out. Often these behaviours occur in apparently normal living environments, which nevertheless are experienced by the child (or dog) as unsafe. The parallels in Saydee's behaviour to those of my patients were confronting.

In Bowlby's (ibid) writing on separation, anger and anxiety, he discusses the likelihood of a fearful and anxious response to the threat of actual harm and how that response is replicated even when it is unlikely harm will occur. It did not matter what I did behaviourally to create safety for Saydee, her response was always the same. I often experience the same phenomenon when using CBT with clients to help them feel safe using strategies. At a very early stage of development, as mammals we can internalise the fear associated with many situations and that that fear will not budge with a strategy.

In Bowlby's (ibid) exploration of mammals and their avoidance of danger, he discusses how animals will not only remain in areas that are familiar and that meet their needs, such as for food, water, climate and safety, but will also narrow that area down to a relatively small and familiar locale. It is only when the basic needs in that area are threatened that the animals will move further afield. He is clear also about how remaining close to that which sustains and keeps the animals physically safe also influences the regulation of the vulnerable young and how this sphere of safety plays a vital role in the psychological state of the dependant. I was therefore resigned to the prospect that I may never be able to assist Saydee in a life totally free from anticipated and perceived fear, with anxious behaviours, just as I might not be able to do with a patient.

Watching her behaviour, I also began to wonder if I was overly optimistic about patient outcomes. One patient, enraged and lacking trust in our work, which was carried out from within a stark psychoanalytic frame which she felt replicated her life with her own absent mother, once accused me of needing 'a crisis in faith' in the psychotherapeutic process. This response was possibly precipitated by the failure of an earlier psychotherapeutic treatment with another practitioner and by her doubt in my capacity to help her. It was not until my practice work began to shift as a result of my exposure to, and integration of, a relational sensibility that we were able to dialogue about both her experiences of her previous practitioner and her experience of the barrenness she felt as a patient within that purist psychoanalytic frame with me. I felt the accusation of that client might have been stimulated by Mitchell's (1988, p. 295) description of the analyst as a *'coactor'* in the patient's drama, in the case of this patient, a drama from all aspects of her developmental life, in which the psychoanalytic frame had created the circumstances for an enactment with me as her unavailable mother. In light of my work with such patients, I had begun to question the wisdom of Saydee's adoption – not so much for me, but for her (and by deduction, my evaluations about some of my patients). Was I capable of giving her (or them) the attachment experience she required to recover? Would I become the object that Saydee (or they) still feared and thus disable my ability to influence her much needed recovery? Fairbairn (1952) explains how the patient forces the psychotherapist to occupy that patient's *antilibidinal state*, a state that has had a rejecting experience through an experience of a neglectful and abusive (parental) home. As the antilibidinal ego is obsessed and consumed at the early stage of child (puppy) development, the resilience of the psychotherapist/dog mother would need to be potent.

In an attempt to create a safe environment, I did find myself tiptoeing around my own life after her arrival. Simple things were done with more care and thought, like emptying the dishwasher, putting cutlery away, opening the saucepan drawer, not slamming bin lids, closing doors and more, in the hope that she might begin to integrate her post-traumatic development and start to feel safe in her present home. For me, it was an interesting time as I noted how much calmer I felt moving about my home more slowly, more deliberately, about being more thoughtful when moving things and doing things. I too had begun to slow down, in harmony with our environment. Using neuroscience, Schore (2015) reconsiders the Winnicottian (1960) notion that there is no baby without a mother, in his consideration of the psychobiological structure supporting socioemotional functioning at the earliest stages of development. He discusses how the growth and development of the infant's brain occur in direct correlation with its environment and explains how the parenting process is both affected by and impacts upon the infant, creating its self-regulatory capacity. I hoped this was occurring with Saydee.

As with patients, it took me quite some time to learn the depth and complexity of the issues Saydee presented and was struggling with. Adding to a long list of those emotional symptoms, there were also many physical concerns. Physically, it was obvious she had not learnt how to eat properly because when she arrived, she was exceedingly thin and was somewhat averse to eating healthy dog food. Her tiny legs had little muscle mass and when I ran my fingers over them, I could feel the bony structure bulging from beneath the thin layer of skin, unprotected by the muscle I knew she needed to avoid sarcopenia as she aged. The major weight-bearing bones, and her little joints, already felt significantly vulnerable without adequate muscle. Around this time, I began frequently thinking about a patient with osteomalacia (previously referred to as rickets) who had a history of severe domestic violence. As with Saydee, it had become imperative that we attend to his physical health issues as much as his psychological issues. While this had been a complex and often problematic journey, at the time of termination we had obtained a satisfactory physical outcome for him. I had once traversed this territory and I guessed that I could again.

Urgency became a factor as Saydee was now three years old, with the muscle mass of a tiny puppy. If she were to lead an injury-free life, we needed to make routine changes, rapidly. I began a boot-camp-style exercise regime and unlike some human participants (including the patient mentioned), Saydee took to her new programme with zeal. While the patient was sent off to a local, well-known trainer, I became Saydee's personal trainer. On one of these early outings, I was disturbed to discover that she did not know how to run. The moment I let her off the lead she would run, inordinately fast, her part-Cavalier ears flying like joyous flags, trying to stay attached to her head in her lightning speed. I noted, with some disbelief, however, that she kept falling over. I was incredulous that a dog could fall over while running. Having grown up on a farm, watching cattle dogs run very fast over long distances, I had not ever seen a dog fall over while running. In fact, I had not ever seen a dog fall over. While her falls were sometimes simple stumbles, frequently they were full and complete tumbles. As impossible as this was to believe, from the little I knew of her history of having grown up in a back garden filled with a swimming pool and pavers, I could surmise that she may never have had the opportunity to run, perhaps rarely, if ever, having been taken out to run in a park, or perhaps even for a walk. Though not deterred now, tail always wagging, tongue hanging out, she would jump up and keep running, at full capacity. After about eight to nine months of her exercise routine, I observed discernible growth in her muscle mass. Simultaneously I noted she fell much less often. To date, she might still stumble and perhaps only occasionally fall when in full flight.

Another symptom, suggestive perhaps of an incomplete intrapsychic developmental process, or of trauma, was Saydee's dislike of water. Teaching her to swim became a part of her recovery treatment plan, while at the same time was an attempt to give her a full range of 'dog-life' experiences, much as I might have done with a human patient's treatment plan. Saydee's usual routine while at the beach would be, barking loudly to intermittently run up to me, just clear of the water's edge to where I had waded. She came to love the beach but was having no part of the water. It clearly evoked some traumatic fear. Later I was to learn why this was so. I knew this turf well. I had had my own water phobia until my late 20s. I knew my fear stemmed from a frequently narrated family story, from which I became vicariously traumatised, in contrast to Saydee's experiential water trauma and phobia. Mine was a story of an uncle, who had only just immigrated to Australia, following other family members to this land of opportunity and new experiences. One glorious summer day he was put in very deep water, with a floatation device he had no idea how to manoeuvre. As it slipped from his grasp he began to flail, then panicking he became submerged. Fortunately for all concerned, an observant bystander recognised the gesticulations of a drowning citizen and fished him out. Though true, this story has been recounted as a jolly family fable in which I still find no humour. Hence my deep respect for Saydee's reticence. When I told Saydee's rescuers about her dislike of water, they told me a story, relayed to them by her departing previous owner as he left on a business trip from which he never returned: 'Oh of course Saydee would hate water; my ex-wife used to randomly toss her in the pool and someone would have to dive in to get her'.

On one particular, relatively warm day on our beach walk, I was lured into the swell, though remaining in the shallows with Saydee looking on. While she watched she paced and barked, paced and barked, paced and barked. I called her name, knowing she loathed not joining in a game. But this game meant water, getting wet, and she was having none of it. Her anxiety was palpable. I was always vigilant not to push her, much as with a patient, when exploring fear and unfamiliar territory and activities. Rothschild (2000) talks about not pushing patients into traumatic material until they are emotionally equipped to manage their ability to recall, and be back in touch with, their trauma. 'With judicious application of the brakes to gradually relieve the pressure, the whole process of trauma therapy becomes less risky' (p. 80). It became imperative that I use this same process with Saydee. I knew if she were ever to find her way into the water, she would do so in her own time again, much like patients; it does not matter how often we 'tell' the patient, change is created by their own awareness that develops over time. I pondered that with children and patients our anxiety to get them to a certain phase can and will undermine their progress. I also knew that she, like many patients, might never find a way into the water, such was her/their traumatic experiences. It was a curious waiting game, as might have been the case with a child learning a new behaviour or a patient exploring their history in the psychotherapy setting. Then, one random beautiful autumn weekend we were down on the south coast of New South Wales, a location where even the most water-phobic person could find something inviting. I ran from the stairway leading down to the beach, straight into the water, the heat of summer receding, though still warm enough for a dip. As I launched myself into the water I looked down and there she was, right on my heels, in the water. With smallish waves splashing about us, I crouched down and played with her. She was barking, running to and fro, frolicking in the water as it lapped her belly, without doing anything specific at that moment she had triumphed over another trauma-related phobia. In terms of change, Lasker (2000) identifies that

> both Bowlby and Kohut acknowledge the crucial role of the psychotherapist in the provision of a safe, secure therapeutic environment from which the patient can explore their life and all its aspects, including relationship biases and the relationship between each other, the impact of the patient's history on their current perceptions and how appropriate or otherwise these may be (p. 7).

It appeared Saydee had traversed some such security in her life with me.

As a reflection of that day I was left wondering whether, if at the moment, she even knew she was in the water or had she prevailed over so many other traumas that the water phobia was no longer a fear. As with patients, there may be change 'without an event' (as one patient often says to me), and that at that moment, Saydee, as happens in the case of patients, may have felt the naturalness of psychological resolution that in turn changes behaviour.

As a psychotherapist and Saydee's mother, I am satisfied with this phase of the treatment.

In the case of Saydee's traumatic responses, I have the feeling she has made considerable inroads into what Berne (1980) refers to as 'cure'. This definition of cure has three main elements. The first is a reduction in symptoms, and is evidenced by people noting and commenting socially on change in the patient; the second is where the patient has introjected the psychotherapist; and the third is where the patient's developing awareness of their own unconscious process becomes more apparent to them and includes overt observable change. I am never lulled into a false sense of security around Saydee's recovery, however, as something as simple as dropping a pen will still have her scuttling off to find safety from the perceived threat, much like us humans. If a patient had reported such a development, it would certainly feel like a psychological change. In terms of Berne's (ibid) 'cure', Saydee had not only had a reduction in symptoms, but it had been noted by others as well as myself that she had had overt observable change. From that day on Saydee has never been afraid of beach water. She will go into the ocean, quite deeply for a height-challenged dog, especially in my company.

At this point in our treatment plan, the majority and immediacy of the trauma responses were relieved enough for us to relax into a harmonious life where we settled into a normal routine. Saydee learns how to hang out with people and other dogs, to ride in the car, go to the shops and much more. She is a polite, well-socialised and well-adjusted canine unless something goes crash, or people raise their voices.

Once my concern about these more overt issues with Saydee began to subside, I noticed other interesting phenomena. I noticed, for example, her reaction to people sneezing. When anyone sneezed Saydee would exhibit an exaggerated startle response, depicting significant distress. She would sit up if she had been lying down or appear from nowhere (by then, she had begun to tolerate being out of my sight) and stare for long periods of time, shrinking and trembling, but always staring, not taking her eyes off the person who sneezed, as if waiting. I would stare back, waiting. Her response was puzzling. Eventually, I would go to her, pick her up and hug her, explaining that it was only sneezing, simulating sneezing in a playful gesture, attempting to familiarise her with it and calm her nervous system.

One day, and I will never really know why, perhaps I was falling into some sort of sync with the trauma patterns of this dog, but all the pieces fell into place. It was like an epiphany. I was sitting up in bed reading, she was dozing nearby, I began staring at her. Many thoughts were stirred and flashed through my mind around her story and our tumultuous time together. I guess in hindsight at some level a part of me was still in the treatment planning phase. I began imagining what it must have been like to live in that house, for any person, especially a dog and a child (there had, in fact, been a child in the house until she, too, was rescued), living in such violence. I began thinking about my patient who grew up in not dissimilar circumstances, a volatile violent home. At that moment I recalled that Saydee's previous owners had been drug users, by their own admission, cocaine having been the drug of choice. I wondered if Saydee had correlated a series of events, just as she had done with many others – in our lives together, for example, lip balm and sunglasses usually meant a walk. According to this theory, was sneezing a prelude to violence? In my practice, I frequently work with cocaine users. The early days of my practice brought with it an interest in this area. In those days I researched and read much about such drug use and its symptoms especially to better assess patients while they were withdrawing. It was often cocaine use that brought people to my rooms. Cocaine was of particular interest to me due to the lack of overt, early side effects. This research revealed a plethora of information on the subject; nose-related symptoms top the list. Cocaine and sneezing cohabit. It would appear that, in Saydee's former home, around the time of sneezing, yelling and arguing would likely have intensified into physical and verbal violence which usually progressed to smashing the home and contents, to axing furniture, and on one occasion, axing every panel of a luxury car, smashing cabinets full of crystal, photo frames, trashing cupboards, anything in their path (behaviour reported by the neighbours who would eventually rescue Saydee and give her up to me for adoption). Drug use escalated violence. At that moment, in bed, it dawned on me. No wonder she had been staring at sneezers. She was waiting for us to turn into the familiar human monster, the unpredictable beast that could love in one moment, then unleash madness in the next. While the phenomenon of her weird staring at sneezing people is no longer a mystery in our life together, it still holds a tight rein over her response to anyone sneezing, perhaps not to be transformed, if we consider the consistency and degree of violence in her previous home.

I was unable to escape the constant reflection on how it must be for traumatised children, and people generally, living in violent homes. Living with Saydee was and always is a stark reminder. It leaves me thinking about how much thought and care it takes to create safety, and how many of our patients might not have had that privilege. This little dog was giving me a first-hand experience of what growing up and living in what often appears externally to be a 'normal' middle-class home and how greatly these events impact children and others, creating the early lives that eventually bring those children, as adults, into our consulting rooms.

This little dog was also teaching me that as much as her trauma occurred in relationship with her previous owners, so does the potential for healing reside within our relationship. Bowlby (1969) contends that the behavioural patterns we develop come unquestionably from how we develop our mental abilities with our early main carers and how we are in relationship. He emphasises that the infant's overarching desire is proximity to its main carers and that if this is attained at an early enough stage and with consistency a healthy developmental attachment will parallel a healthy psychological state. When this does occur, the child, can and will recover and reattach, as has Saydee. Bowlby (ibid) also suggests that a child separated for longer than tolerable periods, or with a mother in unfamiliar and uncomfortable environments, is unable to recover and reattach. In my care, Saydee has not reexperienced the trauma of separation, of 'protesting the missing mother' (Bowlby, 1973) or of despairing that she will never return. With consistent mothering from her human mother, Saydee has shown me how recovery is made possible. She has, in the process, also taught me about patients in the therapeutic setting.

Note

1 This chapter has been adapted from *Delving Deeper: Understanding Diverse Approaches While Exploring Psychotherapy* by Jo Frasca, self-published in 2016.

References

American Psychiatric Association. (1994) *DSM-III: Diagnostic and statistical manual of mental disorders.* Washington, DC: American Psychiatric Association.

Berne, E. (1980) *Transactional analysis in psychotherapy.* London: Souvenir Press.

Bowlby, J. (1969) *Attachment and loss, Volume 1: Attachment.* London: Hogarth Press and the Institute of Psychoanalysis.

Bowlby, J. (1973) *Attachment and loss, Volume 2: Separation, anger and anxiety.* London: Hogarth Press and the Institute of Psychoanalysis.

Fairbairn, W.R.D. (1952) *Psychoanalytic studies of the personality.* London: Routledge & Kegan Paul.

Frances, A. (2013) *The new crisis of confidence in psychiatry diagnosis.* Annals of Internal Medicine, American College of Psychiatrists, acponline.org. Accessed 03/02/2020.

Greenberg, G. (2010) *Manufacturing depression: The secret history of a modern disease.* New York: Simon & Schuster.

Greenberg, G. (2013) *The book of woe: The DSM and the unmaking of psychiatry.* New York: Blue Rider Press Penguin Group.

Lasker (Silbert), J. (2000) *"No man is an island": A comparison between the relational theories of Heinz Kohut and John Bowlby.* Unpublished.

Mitchell, S. (1988) *Relational concepts in psychoanalysis: An integration.* Cambridge, MA and London, UK: Harvard University Press.

Reese, H. (2013) The real problems with psychiatry. *The Atlantic – Health*, https://www.theatlantic.com/health/archive/2013/05/the-real-problems-with-psychiatry/275371/. Accessed 03/11/19.

Rothschild, B. (2000) *The body remembers: The psychophysiology of trauma and treatment.* New York: WW Norton & Company, Inc.

Schore, A.N. (2015) *Affect regulation and the origin of the self: The neurobiology of emotional development.* London and New York: Taylor & Frances Group.

Winnicott, D.W. (1960) The theory of the parent-infant relationship. *International Journal of Psychoanalysis*, 41, pp. 585–595.

9 Sister moon

Close encounters with a third

Gaiana Germani

When I rescued my dog, I considered bringing her to work, but was deterred by the difficulty of finding a pet-friendly office. Years later, stressful events arose, which made it necessary for her to accompany me to work. The successful integration of my dog into my practice was my only path forward. This chapter describes how I did so and how my patients made use of her to heal.

She was a complicated dog with a history of trauma of unknown cause, which was most evident when eager strangers reached out to pet her in the college town where I practice. She was a yellow labrador retriever with the warm soulful eyes of a hound. Her allure was beguiling, but the approaches of strangers were triggers for her. Head and tail lowered, a cautious backward retreat behind my legs, peering between, keeping her eyes on potential dangers. I was her 'haven of safety' (Harlow, 1958, p. 678).

We are unaware of the complex nature of our desire to engage a dog until the interaction does not transpire as we hope. It is an opportunity for others to bear witness to one's goodness, as evidenced by a dog's enthusiastic reception. An anxious mediator during these complex relational events, I aimed to both appease the stranger and protect my dog. 'She's shy,' I would say, or 'She has a history of trauma'. They were offerings, opportunities to gracefully disengage uninjured. Many approached, nonetheless. As if in slow motion, I observed a transformation. Beaming with desire, the strangers' advances were met with my dog's fear hastening their departure, licking their wounded souls. Unencumbered by the compulsion to repeat, she languished not in conflicts from the past; she needs to only avoid them in her present.

My dog was not an ideal candidate for a psychotherapy office – she was not a therapy dog – but our circumstances left us little choice. My colleagues disapproved. They hypothesized that I could not bear separating from my dog, that my relationship with her was 'symbiotic', or that I would be distracted by my desire to gratify her appeal for attention. While it impacted me, I tried to ignore the uninvited commentary. Our circumstances were unknown to them, and my dog rarely sought attention. We lived parallel lives.

First, I found an office with several easily cordoned off nooks for her to hide and rest. I placed a dog bed outside of my peripheral vision, but in the same space as my patients and I, should she want company. Second, I rather rigidly adhered to an edict not to look at her unless my patients called upon me to engage her with them. Third, I developed a protocol for introductions to give patients who wanted to interact with her the best chance of relational success. I instructed patients to enter the room quietly, avert their gaze, sit on the couch, and hold their hands low, palms up with a biscuit invitation.

Once I formulated the logistics, designed a protocol for introductions, coped with my colleagues' opinions, and contemplated the character of our dyad, I turned toward the literature I hoped would illuminate the theoretical implications of bringing a dog to a psychotherapy office. One article discussed home offices, which I believed raised similar issues as bringing a dog to work. The author used phrases like: 'overstimulated... by personal information ... flood ... overwhelming ... analyst hunger to be known ... fill a void ... forcing ... sadistic ... malignant regression ...' (Maroda, 2007, pp. 174–176) – not unlike my colleagues' concerns. I panicked. I could not afford to shake my confidence. I set the article aside and decided instead to lean on giants such as Sigmund Freud, Anna Freud, Frieda Fromm Reichman, Harry Stack Sullivan, Karen Horney, Melanie Klein, and Lewis Aron, each of whom allowed their dogs into their psychotherapy offices. If they managed the boundaries, then perhaps I could as well. I also committed myself to an open-minded, keen-eyed hypervigilance in my triadic practice. Not quite oxymoronic, but one suggests ease and the other anxiety.

Sister moon and Saint Francis of Assisi: a song, a dog, and the artist change the analyst

A religious man began our analysis with a vow of silence hoping to hear from God. A quiet dyad awaiting a third. As if by a miracle, upon introduction, my dog was unusually at ease and affectionate. A fast, mutual bond formed between them. Breaking his vow, he gave us the blessing of new Christian names. He pointed to her and then to me and said, 'Sister Moon and Mother Earth'. I later explored Saint Francis of Assisi's 'Canticle of Creatures' (1999) and after reading the poem, I embraced our new names. Assisi's Sister Moon is 'clear' and 'precious' (Assisi, p. 114). Clear because she is unconflicted about reality, precious because she could offer that wisdom to us. Assisi's Mother Earth 'sustains and governs us, and produces various fruits, coloured flowers, and herbs' (ibid, p. 114). I nurture my patients and I govern the frame, a job now challenged with the addition of my dog. Creating meaning in complex transitions holds us together in times of uncertainty and distress. The name 'Sister Moon' was an affirming talisman holding the promise of the clarity it evokes.

A miracle perhaps, but the uncanny was also in play. I often referred to her as the moon in my orbit. Ever present, but aloof.

Sister moon and the FBI

Patients often broke with protocol, and Siros was no exception. Siros was sixty when we met. Relentlessly depressed and profoundly alone in the world, he was unable to chart a course to connectedness. His childhood home was rife with violence and abandonment. Often extracted, he was helpless in the current of social services, drowning in a sea of his peers without a safe harbour. As an adult, his efforts to connect were invariably met with rejection. Afterwards, a fog descended for days until the lucid awareness of his loneliness emerged, lurching forward, penetrating his deadening depression giving rise to a soulful howling agony swallowed whole and replaced by fantasies of being followed by the FBI – one of the psyche's cruellest solutions to loneliness (Michalska da Rocha et al., 2017).

Siros was thrilled by the prospect of meeting Sister Moon. I, on the other hand, never having witnessed Siros's transition from socially hopeful, to rejection, to psychosis, was apprehensive.

Our hour arrived, and I pantomimed, 'do not look, sit down, palms up and low, never approach from above', and so on before we entered the office. Siros instantaneously abandoned protocol. He looked directly at her with enthusiasm, gesticulating wildly, encouraging her to come near his hand darted out to pat the top of her head. She instinctually ducked and backed away quickly to her corner of the room. She was not a welcoming mirror reflecting his desire to be received (Winnicott, 1953). Sister Moon's boundaries were clear, and recovery was dubious. I gently reminded Siros of the steps. Hands low, palms up, look away. Eventually, she gave him a second chance, accepted a biscuit from him, and a tentative scratch under her ear. Eventually, like with most of my patients, a natural rhythm evolved. After some mutual affection, Sister Moon lazily returned to her dreamscapes.

One concern I harboured regarding the introduction protocol was that it had the potential to be a re-enactment of the submissive stance adopted by Siros to keep himself safe while seeking comfort from family members. However, Sister Moon's requirement for introductory submission was not cut from the same cloth. This submission liberated her, creating space into which their shared desire could expand. The submission required by his family was sadistically intended to dominate and scare him. Compliance was the price he paid for affection as a child. It was not real, but it was better than nothing, just like the FBI.

The submission Sister Moon required allowed them both to move towards a safe, authentic, and mutually gratifying connection. If Winnicott (1969) observed the encounter, he might define the unfolding of events as an example of 'good enough' (ibid, p. 712) mothering, providing the safety of a holding environment in which two separate beings meet having become real for each other. The office space, the protocol, my guidance, and Sister Moon's prerequisites, all components of a holding environment, made a developmental shift in Siros possible. Winnicott would describe this shift as 'object relating' to 'object usage' (ibid, p. 712). Siros was able to experience her as other than him. They shared reality as two separate beings. I believe Siros needed both Mother Earth's governing (the protocol) and Sister Moon's clarity (instinctually and incontrovertibly real, she can be nothing other than her nature) for the evolution of this shift. And while there was indeed a re-enactment of sorts, Sister Moon's need for submission and his capacity to meet that need in a healing rather than sadistic context was what Dowd might have called a 'repetition with a difference' (2016, p. 7).

Sister Moon is not a miracle worker, and correlation is not causation, but, gradually, Siros experienced some social success in his community, joining people for meals, and sharing community spaces.

The FBI was less and less a presence in his life.

After meetings with Sister Moon, he revealed he lived his life thinking his only hope for belonging and love was to find a way to be an 'entirely different person.' A tragic Winnicottian 'false self' (Winnicott, 1955, p. 21).

Siros learned with Mother Earth and Sister Moon that even a small shift in social behaviour could make a substantial difference. He need not change everything about himself to connect.

Phantasmagorical sister moon

Anath struggled to connect the depth of her despair to her experiences growing up in her family. 'But nothing bad ever happened to me', a neglected child's near-universal refrain. The steam of her parents' open sexuality and audible encounters, the promised crack of a baseball bat kept at her father's bedside to murder inevitable intruders and the stench of mouldy clothing left to dry in the washer by her mother was the atmosphere Anath breathed as a child.

When I met Anath, she suffered devastating panic attacks accompanied by prolific paranoid thoughts of being followed by murderous men looking for the right moment to strike.

Her 'baseball bat' was her vivid imagination replacing intrusive thoughts of imminent murder with fantasies of safety and power. She kept pictures of Sister Moon and I open on her computer monitors at work. She was able to pull herself away from panicked states and paranoid thoughts with Sister Moon and me near.

The phantasmagorical imagination of Anath represented both her conscious desire to be safe in the world while simultaneously illuminating the rage she split off to keep safe her mind. One fantasy featured Sister Moon and me. Below, is the narrative as I remember it from that day:

> As a warrior goddess with long blond hair flowing aft in the vespers, I walk before her, wielding a sword, Sister Moon at my side. She and I both radiate and exist in a magical golden flowing light trailing our

course. Anath is entrapped in a blue glow holding her captive as she walks behind us. Sometimes she is able to free herself from the grip of the blue glow and take steps forward toward Sister Moon and me. When she does, she is enveloped by our dreamy golden atmosphere, leaving the blue behind her awaiting her inevitable return. In the golden light, I am at her command, and as my commander, she tells me to kill unhesitatingly and without question, anyone she thinks would bring us to harm.

Sister Moon's role was complex. As a loyal vessel, she contained the love and warmth Anath received from me, which was unavailable during imagined homicidal rampages. Sister Moon was there to 'bear witness' to my atrocities, so I would not be 'alone' as I carried out Anath's murderous commands. Lastly, she was to guard my imago, which would be necessarily split off from the traumatising horror of what transpired. Sister Moon contained, guarded, and protected what I would need to reintegrate and return the whole woman Anath counted on outside of the golden glow.

Anath's fantasy evokes a thicket of theory. I will clear one path. Heinz Kohut believed that 'agoraphobia resulted from maternal failures to function adequately as an idealised self-object, and, in this developmental context, to provide sufficient calming and soothing means of preventing anxiety from spreading and reaching "panicked states"' (Miliora and Unman, 1996, p. 220). Anath was unable to utilise her mother as a self-object. However, she made use of Sister Moon and me as an idealised self-object pair providing 'the experience of merger [stepping into the golden glow] with the calm, power, wisdom, and goodness of idealised persons' (Moore and Fine, 1990). She needed a mother who could remain intact and protect her from the savage in her home. Sister Moon, Mother Earth and Anath were the triad necessary for her 'developmental second chance' (Orange, 1995, p. 4).

Conclusion

Bringing Sister Moon to my office required logistical planning, protocols, and confidence in myself. Though she was not often a central figure for my patients, these vignettes illustrate the power of her presence when patients made use of Sister Moon to heal. For Siros, she offered the authentic responding to realise he need not change his whole self to relate. Anath called upon Sister Moon to hold our psyches together while she located the rage, which once integrated, will make her the powerful, unstoppable force of her namesake. In triads of trauma, my dog did the trick.

References

Assisi, F. (1999) The canticle of creatures (Translated by R. Armstrong). In *Francis of Assisi: Early Documents. Volume 1: The Saint*: R.J Armstrong, J.A.W. Hellman and W.J. Short. (Eds.) New York: New City Press, pp. 35–167.

Dowd, D. (2016) States of grace: A relational context for a patient's coming into being. *Psychoanalytic Dialogues*, 26(5), pp. 564–570.

Harlow, H.F. (1958) The nature of love. *American Psychologist*, 13(12), pp. 673–685.

Maroda, K.J. (2007) Ethical considerations of the home office. *Psychoanalytic Psychology*, 24(1), pp. 173–179.

Michalska da Rocha, B., Rhodes, S., Vasilopoulou, E. and Hutton, P. (2017) Loneliness in psychosis: A meta-analytical review. *Schizophrenia Bulletin*, 44(1), pp. 114–125.

Miliora, M.T. and Ulman, R.B. (1996) Panic disorder: A bioself-psychological perspective. *Journal of the American Academy of Psychoanalysis*, 24(2), pp. 217–256.

Moore, B.E. and Fine, B.D. (1990) *Psychoanalytic terms and concepts*. New Haven, CT: Yale University Press.

Orange, D.M. (1995) *Emotional understanding: Studies in psychoanalytic epistemology*. New York: Guilford Press.

Winnicott, D.W. (1953) Transitional objects and transitional phenomena; A study of the first not-me possession. *The International Journal of Psychoanalysis*, 34, pp. 89–97.

Winnicott, D.W. (1955) Metapsychological and clinical aspects of regression within the psycho-analytical set-up. *International Journal of Psychoanalysis*, 36, pp. 16–26.

Winnicott, D.W. (1969) The use of an object. *International Journal of Psycho-Analysis*, 50, pp. 711–716.

10 Frame breakage to the rescue[1]

Jo Frasca

Some time ago, with perhaps a combination of inspiration and trepidation from Freud's work, I felt liberated enough to introduce a frowned-upon practice into my psychotherapy room. While Freud did write about his observations of his dogs in the room, he did so without really exploring their role in terms of his own theoretical paradigm. It was with my limited knowledge of this history that I furthered my own daring on the subject.

It is Freud's love of his dogs and the power and status he attributed to them that lead Anna Freud to famously claim that her father had, 'transferred his whole interest in her on to [Anna's dog] Wolf', (Young-Bruehl, 1988, p. 217) and his own comment that 'our Wolf almost replaces the lost Heinerle' (Freud's six-year-old grandson who died of tuberculosis in 1928) (Molnar, 1996, p. 275) that reveals how his dog became a surrogate family member and helped him deal with painful grief. Freud's introduction of his pets into his clinical practice, however, was met with varying degrees of tolerance by his patients. Hilda Doolittle, for example, was somewhat displeased: 'Jofi would 'wander about' at the end of the session and 'the Professor was more interested in Jofi than he was in my story' (Doolittle, 1956, p. 162). Furthermore, Freud's experience of owning a dog would precipitate his decision to end his life. It is documented (Edmundson, 2007; Schur, 1972) that shortly after his beloved dog Lün began howling, repulsed by the smell, and turned away from Freud's necrotic mouth cancer, on 23 September 1939, Freud died from two hypodermic injections, of between 15 and 25 mg of morphine, administered twelve hours apart (Schur, 1972).

Perhaps such accounts speak to Freud's devotion to his pets and may help us understand his decision to bring both the company and the love of his dogs into his practice room. If so, then what is discussed in this chapter will not be such a surprise.

As a result of having learnt something of Freud's accounts of the effect of his dogs on his patients, the psychoanalytic process and his practice, and when the vet insisted that I could not let my own dog, following a serious illness, out of my sight for several weeks, I knew managing this would be a challenge. One never makes a decision to change anything in the therapeutic space without knowing there will be a substantial impact on the therapeutic relationship. I became preoccupied with whether to do so.

I have two practice locations, one in the Sydney Central Business District and another in my home in suburbia. Working from home often interferes with practice routines and as a result, I am frequently challenged with how to manage a frame affected by domestic issues which make working in that environment, not such an ideal option. Occurrences such as garbage day, the mail – or any other – deliveries, the lawn mowing man, and visitors arriving early all create contaminations of the frame – although these events, which I might not otherwise have wished upon psychotherapy patients, do habitually provoke important – and often therapeutically useful – conversations.

My study and my development of the relational model in my practice slowly precipitated significant changes in my thinking and working style. Relational theory fashioned ways in which to discuss such frame disturbances with the patient and offered ways to consider how that rupture inevitably unleashes latent anger, frustrations, or unspoken feelings and experiences. Such conversations helped to create a more solid relational platform from which the patient could work and develop by allowing opportunities that would not have occurred within a more stringent psychoanalytic frame, for discussing relational nuances. Stern (in Aron, Grand, Slochower, 2018, p. 28) writes, 'there is no sense in addressing someone about a sensitive subject unless you communicate in a way that really speaks to that person'.

And now I was to be challenged in my home practice by yet another external factor – the arrival of a highly traumatised, now unwell, rescue dog. I was about to traverse territory that Freud had shone a dim light on, although without having provided us with any clear theoretical direction. I became preoccupied with how bringing Saydee into the therapeutic space might impede my usual way of working and also affect the frame. Such is the importance of the frame that Casement (1990) reminds us that when the analytic space is kept free from influences that could distort or disable it, the process then unfolds and can be trusted and followed. Could I make that quantum leap by bringing a dog into in the therapeutic setting, and still work in a way that was consistent with my psychoanalytic practice, a framework which informed my work for many years? Could I hold that frame, which could be partly devoured by the inclusion of an unpredictable third? Occasionally I had heard my own internal critic's alarm in response to stepping outside the very clear boundary of that psychoanalytic space as Casement outlines. Early on I had been disapproving of the 'unnecessary' inclusion by other practitioners of such things as family snaps and collectibles into the psychotherapeutic space. Was I about to consider a similar faux pas? My question to my peer group as to whether I bring Saydee into my own clinical room was met with scepticism, alarm, and concern. As a result, I was reticent to discuss in much detail with colleagues my experimentally and intentionally breaking the frame by bringing Saydee into the room, fearing that I might suffer similar criticism I had dispensed towards others.

The relational psychotherapy principle of the third, however, provided an alternative perspective for me to consider the introduction of Saydee into my clinical practice. Aron (2006) discusses the flexibility of the relational structure of thirdness in our move away from subject/object, us/them, and moving into thinking about working within a frame that supports the development of clinical work. Benjamin's (2018) notion of *rupture to repair* allows us to think about working with vulnerability and imperfections towards a more collaborative approach between the patient and psychotherapist. The patient's contribution, she argues, enables repair even though repair might occur via their protests. It was this idea that liberated me from my concerns and authorised my bringing Saydee into the room. No matter the protest of the patient, a relational approach provided me with a way of thinking and working with the possible rupture of Saydee's inclusion, and furthermore, it was even likely to benefit the patient – or so I told myself.

Part of the decision to bring Saydee into the therapeutic space was fostered by her first arrival in my home when I had left her in the outer rooms of the house; her separation anxiety was such that she would become persistently noisy if she knew I was within close proximity. She would scratch at the closed-door closest to her, and, in her attempt to remind me of her existence, would bark intermittently. I felt frustration and irritation at this new addition to my world, which complicated and affected all areas of my life. I had become exceedingly aware of, and concerned about, my own agitation while working. I was concerned about how my unexpressed distraction and agitation would unavoidably find its way into the room and be felt unconsciously or otherwise by the patient. In knowing Saydee was nearby and distressed, what would I be affecting and stimulating in the room? Could I be momentarily distracted to the detriment of the patient?

After several sessions with Saydee outside the room, it was evident this arrangement was not working and proved distressing for us both. I began to feel that it would be more unfavourable for the patient to have this traumatised, anxious object outside the room than inside. It fast became apparent that I would need to begin considering more seriously the implications of bringing this damaged little dog into sessions.

I had had two colleagues who had successfully managed to introduce a dog into the clinical environment and as this would not be the first time I had worked with a dog in the therapeutic room, this was somewhat familiar, yet slightly different terrain. Many years earlier, at the beginning of my work as a psychotherapist, my previous dog, Doogie, was already with me in the room when I began to work with my patients – my then patients already knew me with a dog. Doogie developed relationships with certain patients, which is discussed later in this chapter, but Doogie's presence in sessions felt different to what was about to unfold with Saydee; the experience of bringing a new, and traumatised, object in the form of Saydee into an existing relationship felt considerably different.

Also, at the time that I was thinking about introducing Saydee into my practice, I was not taking new patients and each existing patient was long term. Much of my practice was made up of patients who had been diagnosed with varying degrees of attachment disorders. My main therapeutic considerations about bringing Saydee into the room were whether, in spite of my fears and concerns, the likelihood of the protest Benjamin (2018) discusses and the issues the dog might trigger for the patient, I could allow a positive process and outcome to occur.

I felt cautious. I was concerned, in particular, about my borderline patients. With a persistent instability of interpersonal relationships for the borderline personality, which developed through early infant rupture, the internal structures of patients with this type of attachment disorder are inevitably affected by interactions with the psychotherapist. Impulsive reactions are common. Such reactions may emerge in the form of an enactment where the patient moves into a dissociative space reflective of their early traumatic experience and responses. These early experiences have affected the patient's ability to self-regulate thereby compromising their ability to work relationally with the psychotherapist (Bromberg, 2011).

In the occasional caring and nurturing from the borderline or attachment disordered patient towards the psychotherapist, there is a covert, unarticulated agreement lurking. This covert message is a sort-of quid-pro-quo expectation on the part of the patient that the same care and nurturing, or more, will be reciprocated, by the psychotherapist. If the psychotherapist fails to reciprocate in the way the patient desires, rage-fuelled punitive action will invariably follow. With this type of internal processing, and the common associated features of fallacious self-image and acute impulsivity, I knew a dog's presence would likely be a deeply provocative trigger. Fear of rejection, abandonment and separation has an incalculable impact on the self-image, thinking, feelings and behaviour of these patients. The borderline patient has the ability to idealise the psychotherapist in one moment and engage in severe animosity in the next. The exertion of this power is a formidable, often discombobulating experience, even for any veteran practitioner. I feared, though, that it would be much worse for a dog, and a highly traumatised dog at that. This can be a savage attack and I did not want the dog to have a traumatic experience as a result of a decision I had made bringing her into an environment with a patient with borderline features.

The question was not *if* Saydee would impact the relationship, but *how* she would impact the therapeutic relationship, and how I might manage that impact. While I was aware, of course, that Saydee's presence might trigger the patient's archaic wounds which in turn would evoke a plethora of feelings, and that this may offer valuable therapeutic opportunities for us, I was also juggling other feelings of protection towards Saydee – perhaps a three-way countertransferential process: me projecting onto Saydee my concerns for myself and for the fragile relationship with my patients. I also felt concerned about how I might manage the dog's experience when that happened. It brings to light the work of Benjamin (2018), where she relieves the stressors of fearing the rupture of thirdness by considering that we can use this potential power struggle as an opportunity to explore together, with the patient, a mutually beneficial affective outcome.

In spite, or perhaps in view of all of the above, I forged ahead with what I hoped was my well-monitored and well-researched experiment. As a practitioner who works predominantly with transference and countertransference, I felt that I could manage the responses that would predictably find their way into the therapeutic space and that these responses might even allow rich material, as Benjamin (ibid) suggests, to surface, material that otherwise may take years to arrive in the room. Furthermore, I could reverse the decision to have Saydee in the sessions if it became too much for the patients.

So, in many unexpected ways, we began the journey of healing.

Early introductions

N usually attends the home practice where the dog is now firmly ensconced, but on this occasion, she sailed into the practice room in the CBD, where Saydee had not yet been introduced and says, 'How's that dog version of me?' To which I reply, 'She is well thank you'. She sinks into her favourite position on the couch and I ask, 'I wonder what parallels you draw between Saydee and yourself?' Quick as a flash she retorts, 'we both wag our tails when we see you'. I deliberate over this statement a moment, then say, 'I'm not sure you always wag your tail when you see me'.

Pause. Silence. Nothing forthcoming from the patient.

She knows.

I wait, then turn the covert overt and say, 'Last week you threw a cushion at me in anger. Can I assume today you are pleased to be here?' Disliking the reminder of her outburst from last week's session she says, 'Yeah, I'm sorry about last week. Sometimes I hate you and could spit at you; this week I love you'. She beautifully articulates the classic borderline struggle with whether to hate or love the object and how this can vary dramatically from session to session, or even moment to moment.

We discuss how painful this road has been. Her life since thirteen has been an ever-increasing series of deep cuts, cuts with a blade, cuts sometimes requiring anything up to twenty stiches, cuts which she vividly describes as turning 'white, then red, then orange, then yellow' as she slices through her own flesh. She wears scars 'from hate', a hatred directed towards herself, on every limb of her body, barring her right arm. After six years of psychotherapy, she is only just beginning to understand that her self-hatred comes from an interpretation she made as an infant of her experience of an unavailable, violent, angry mother with a mental illness. She has never been able to traverse the topic of 'hate', other than by her overt, self-cutting, though she is slowly beginning to understand that she is enacting what her own mother might have felt towards her.

A wandering mind

A breakthrough came when K attended a third weekly session of her eight years of psychotherapy.

Saydee had begun coughing violently and while I knew enough not to take my attention from the patient, I did want to be sure the dog was not choking to death in the corner of the room. I momentarily diverted my eyes to see what the dog was doing. In that split second of distraction I was condemned and seriously chastised with vehement vitriol. K's tirade pervaded the room. 'I knew you'd be more focused on the fucking dog ... I know you don't even know I'm in the room when the fucking dog is here ... I don't want her here ... get her the fuck out ... I hate you ... I hate that fucking dog'.

There it was. All I had been anticipating from Saydee's entry into the room. Florid. Palpable. Yes, I could have immediately got up and removed the dog from the space. In doing so, however, I would not only have prevented the rich transferential material from being processed but I would also have prevented the regressed and triggered Child ego state (Berne, 1964) from her early developmental thoughts, feelings, and behaviours, from expressing all that was being generated by my attention to Saydee. Had I gratified her demands and removed Saydee at that point, I might have foreclosed on a significant therapeutic opportunity to provide for the patient a space safe enough to effectively renegotiate previously unchartered developmental challenges. The dynamic might have been similar to parents gratifying the unreasonable demands of an uncontrollable two-year-old.

While K's family – mother, father, brother, and grandparents – all tried to kill each other in her young presence, she did what she needed to survive. With that same skill she was going to manage Saydee and I. Somewhere in her archaic experience she knew she had to manage me to protect herself. I knew that for her to recover and lead a full life, it would not be useful for her to be managing every person she encountered. She would need to learn that I am potent enough to manage all that goes on in the room – no matter how much she wanted to push those boundaries. And I would do that with her assistance, rather than her control.

Once the onslaught abated, I waited for quite some time to pass before I responded. I did not break eye contact with her. Finally, I asked, 'Perhaps you fear Saydee will steal my love from you?' Staring back, also maintaining contact with me, her eyes filled. Tears rolled down her cheeks. She nodded. After a few more minutes of silence I added, 'I'm gathering Saydee feels to you like a threat right now.' With her mascara streaming down her face, creating black trails like those seen after the fury of a bushfire and seeping onto the white cushion she was hugging close to her chest, she nodded again. In that moment I saw her in the rubble of her early life, the carnage pulpable. She appeared like the crumpled doll someone had tossed in the corner, limp, hair adrift, a mask of black rivers running down her face. I imagine this might have been how she felt on those dark nights, watching, waiting, hearing them trying to kill each other. It would take only a severe slash into her own flesh to drown that out.

In cases of self-injury, I note that the rate of the recurrence of cutting is always high, when tumultuous feelings reappear. While this might generate fear for the psychotherapist and thus tempt the psychotherapist to intervene to stop the behaviour, I have found it more useful to locate the historical source of the cutting. This patient speaks of killing herself, often. In recent months it has escalated. I also know that if her belief is that I have embedded Saydee into my life, and with a resurgence of those painful feelings of terror, abandonment, and aloneness, death might be the only option she could envisage. Knowing she lacks language when regressed in trauma, more quietly I share my image asking, 'Are you feeling discarded, abandoned?' As if hearing my thinking, she adds, 'Yes, like when they fought.' She shuffled. I wondered if she might speak again. She does, almost inaudibly at first. 'I've been feeling like I finally found someone to see and hear me, somewhere I feel safe and I bet Saydee will take that from me. So I hate her.' Now, finally, we can talk about the hate, not pretend it does not exist.

She finally articulates intense feelings, moving through an impasse, no longer using the defences recruited to avoid the ridicule, rejection and the feelings of insignificance of an earlier stage when her existence and feelings were not validated. Now, if I am thoughtful about the impact that Saydee as a third has in the room she may have the chance to understand and be understood. By giving voice to the protest (Benjamin, 2018) and by using Saydee as her object she is able to say she loves me, following hating me. It is also the first time the patient has been able to overtly express both love and hate. When K understands that I see her, from both my description of her being discarded and asking if she fears loosing me to Saydee, she is able to relive the feeling she had in the room and link them back to a time in her family, now knowing these are not the same in that moment but that they are a stimulation of a dissociated experience (Bromberg, 2011). Bromberg (ibid) asserts that the activation of the dissociated experience in this way is essential for the process to develop and progress. By diverting my eyes onto the dog and my attention away from the patient I had triggered an archaic experience of abandonment and aloneness. After she was able to challenge me about my alliance with Saydee, and after my articulation of her concerns, eventually she was able to understand that my thinking and feeling towards her was not as she experienced in her family.

The dog has facilitated, language, love and hate in the room.

Speechless

On reflection I have wondered if the advent of Saydee's integration into the psychotherapy room was as a result of my previous love, Doogie. Doogie was often described as 'that animal from The Never-Ending Story' or 'an Ewok from Star Wars'; self-declared dog-haters loved Doogie. His warm, loving nature made it easy to integrate him into the space, though Doogie's foray into the therapeutic room was perhaps more by default than as a result of a considered process such as Saydee's introduction was.

A friend had given me a tiny handmade garden post that read *One spoilt dog lives here*. Some family member had randomly stuck it in the garden without thought about its message to any unsuspecting passer-by – quite acceptable unless the homeowner is psychotherapist, working from home.

For some time, I had been working with S who could barely speak due to trauma, which, together with her experience of having been inappropriately parented, compromised her ability to parent her own baby. The combination of her depressive state and her traumatic background also limited our work options. CBT seemed to be the best modality in helping her to develop her life and parenting skills. One day she came into the room with much more vigour than her usual malaise – perhaps even animated, asking 'You have a dog?'. I was so surprised I did not even manage to do the famous psychotherapeutic line, 'What is it that makes you think I have a dog?' Or even more feebly, 'How do you feel about knowing I have a dog?' I just spontaneously, and in hindsight intuitively, said, 'Yes I do.' She had seen the sign in the garden. Shyly she said, 'I love dogs'. Then, as if I did not hear, or did not hear the importance of what she was saying, she said, in an almost childlike manner,

> very, very, much. I walk and look after a dog now and again for this old man who lives near me. He struggles to walk, so I help him with things. I love walking his dog the best. Can I meet your dog?

Mild alarm coursed through my body, plagued by the caution 'the frame, do not break the frame'. My tentativeness in that moment might have appeared to be matched by her own tentativeness. In my case, however, my response related to my fear of a frame breakage, though it could have been interpreted by the patient as a well-considered and thoughtful; in hindsight a sort of mirroring of this patient's usual mood.

The therapeutic space being invaded by something other than the patient and the psychotherapist or the effect of a frame breakage, is always a concern. While it might appear to be a good idea in the moment, mostly it is not. Usually we are left to mop up a gory, emotional mess with the patient at some later stage. A patient once accused me (in that tone) of fearing a frame breakage to protect myself, not her. Perhaps there is some truth in that. Those gory, messy sessions are hard work and the repercussions can reverberate for years. However, the words 'do no harm' are also in our charter, and I felt a dog visit fell into that category for this patient. This day, therefore, I heard myself say, with more calm that I actually felt, 'Yes of course you can meet my dog. His name is Doogie.'

I went to the door of the consulting room, which opens off into the main part of the house and called his name, knowing he would be close by. He knew these people who visited his home. He had been familiar with their voices, their stories, their smell, their distress, their footsteps and probably much more which only a dog might know, as is in keeping with dog responsibilities. As I called his name this day, he was there at the door, in a flash, though initially he would go no further than the threshold; to date he had only been allowed in this space when it was patient-free. Briefly I wondered if he was even more reticent than S or I. Because she wanted to meet him, I forged on, giving him the go-ahead nod. He went straight to her and lay at her feet, not mine – as if this was a normal thing to do, as if this was something he did every day, something they shared regularly. I was surprised to observe her slide off the couch onto the floor near him, wriggling into a position as close to him as possible without disturbing his selected space. She immediately began stroking him. This would be the position they remained in for the rest of that session, and the position they assumed in her sessions from that day forward. Looking at them together, it appeared that this had been prearranged between them, so natural was their bond.

The remarkable thing about the change in the room was how her session content transformed from that day forward. Henceforth, each session began with a greeting to Doogie, and a question about how he was and what he had been up to. Sometimes S would give him a little rendition of her week, which was ever-so informative to the psychotherapist. This was more than I had ever been able to extract from those lips. Woollams and Brown (1979) use the *carom* as a metaphor to describe an attempt, conscious or unconscious, at communication, where one person's intention (S, in this instance) is to impel a message off to the second person (Doogie) onto a third (me), which is for whom the real transmission of information was intended, as happens with the balls in the game of billiards. A carom in billiards, when used at the right time, is an important, formidable shot, whereby the cue ball ricochets into another ball, using the second ball to shoot another (the intended) ball into the pocket. There may be some parallels between the notion of the carom and the relational concept of the third. Benjamin (in Mitchell and Aron, 1999) refers to the two experiences that the patient has: that of recognising the psychotherapist as a part of their own inner world and also as a part of another – in a way the intrapsychic and intersubjective aspects of relating. This allows not only the opportunity for relating where that has been difficult, but also at another level allows that exploration of both feelings and relating without the threat of direct engagement. The psychological significance here is that as this patient had used mutism as a defence; it had become too difficult for her to communicate directly to another human, or adult. A canine, however, was less threatening and allowed that communication without risk. Whether conscious or unconscious in this case, S was so engrossed in her dialogue with Doogie it was almost as if my role was superfluous. Thereafter I began to hear all sorts of things offered as information to Doogie, which would drive our work forward into uncharted territory.

In breaking the frame, and allowing a third into the therapeutic space, the patient was able to liberate her voice, then her story, into a non-threatening third allowing us to work within that space, so as to progress something greater than the two of us had been able to achieve.

Note

1 This chapter has been adapted from *Delving Deeper: Understanding Diverse Approaches While Exploring Psychotherapy* by Jo Frasca, self-published in 2016.

References

Aron, L. (2006) Analytic impasse and the third: Clinical implications of intersubjectivity theory. *International Journal of Psychoanalysis*, 87(2), pp. 349–368.

Aron, L., Grand S. and Slochower, J. (2018) *Decentring relational theory: A comparative critique*. Oxon: Routledge.

Benjamin, J. (2018) *Beyond doer and done to*. London and New York: Routledge.

Berne, E. (1964) *Games people play*. New York: Grove Press.

Bromberg, P. (2011) *The shadow of the tsunami: And the growth of the relational mind*. New York and Oxon: Routledge.

Casement, P. (1990) *Further learning from the patient: The analytic space and process*. London: Routledge.

Doolittle, H. (1956) *A tribute to Freud*. Boston: Godline.

Edmundson, M. (2007) *The death of Sigmund Freud: The legacy of his last days*. New York: Bloomsbury.

Mitchell, S A. and Aron, L. (1999) *Relational psychoanalysis: The emergence of a tradition*. New York and London: Routledge.

Molnar, M. (1996) Of dogs and doggerel. *American Imago*, 53(3), pp. 269–280.

Schur, M. (1972) *Freud: Living and dying*. New York: International Universities Press.

Woollams, S. and Brown, M. (1979) *The total handbook of transactional Analysis*. Upper Saddle River, NJ: Prentice Hall.

Young-Bruehl, E. (1988) *Anna Freud: A biography*. New York: Summit Books.

11 A cat in the clinical hour

Gretchen Heyer

Rituals of frame

A Sufi story tells of a cat that belongs to one of the Sufi masters rubbing against seated meditators, interrupting their focus. The solution becomes to tie the cat up during meditation. But the cat lives a long time, and the Sufi master dies. Younger monks continue to tie up the cat during meditation, and by the time the cat dies people have forgotten why the cat was tied up in the first place, and so buy another cat to tie it up for meditation (Shah, 1988).

This story highlights the dynamics of ritual, community memory, and the actual restraining of a cat – dynamics at the heart of this paper. I am exploring the impact of a cat I restrained during a patient's clinical hour and the way this touched pre-oedipal issues in the transference/countertransference, as well as providing a symbolic bridge through cultural hatreds of racism filled with malevolence and violence.

Among the rituals of psychoanalysis and psychotherapy, the clinical hour is one of the most significant and enduring. The hour is framed by time and walls, by the couch and chairs in which people sit, by objects in the room, as well as silences and words within that hour. The frame of the clinical hour is of importance because it provides a space where the outside is separated from the inside, so the inside can better be attended to.

Yet, inside and outside are never completely separate, and the intrusions become as important as the frame itself. The clinical hour is intruded upon when airplanes fly overhead, family members die or become ill, lawns are mowed, hurricanes strike, the patient brings in ice-cream and the analyst's own mind wanders. The traditional clinical hour was first and foremost a ritual of words, with nonverbal communication translated into words. But now intrusions and enactments, actions and objects, can be seen as communications in their own right, rather than resistance disrupting the course of a therapeutic process. The analyst is no longer merely abstaining, remaining neutral to avoid gratifying instinctive drives, but can be an active participant. In the early years of the psychoanalytic relational movement, Stephen Mitchell observed the move away from word interpretations exclusively, towards the inclusion of objects and actions, to be rooted in a shift of understanding humans as meaning-generating animals rather than primarily drive regulated (1993).

But if the ritual frame of the clinical hour becomes one where intrusions are valued as much as words, where enactments are intrinsic to the process, a greater responsibility is required of the analyst to question what is occurring for the symbolic and metaphorical meaning it holds.

Ava and I

Enactment intrusions wove into my work with Ava from the beginning when my mind began a pattern of shutting down. Within minutes of our meeting, Ava asked if I was Christian. It is not my usual practice to answer personal questions without understanding where the questions come from, but it seemed Ava spoke of how we needed to connect, wanting a clear, spoken link. I flashed through ways to respond as if I had to give a complete and factual answer. I no longer described myself as Christian, but what roots did I have if they were not Christian? I answered 'yes'. Ava then asked if I was 'saved by the blood of Jesus Christ'. 'As a child,' I said. But suddenly anxious at this representation of myself, I rushed on to say I did not work as any sort of Christian counsellor. 'Whatever', Ava said, waving her hand through the air. 'I can see you're not black and I hope you're not prejudiced, but if you and I don't share Christianity, I don't know how this can work.'

Screaming fights and the taut, angry silence between her parents punctuated Ava's childhood. Her father worked two, often three jobs. He also engaged in public affairs with multiple women in the community. When she discovered the affairs, Ava's mother refused to clean or cook, often never leaving the house. Little Ava cleaned and cooked. In the evenings when her father came home, he praised her for this, while her mother hated and envied her, striking her physically as well as verbally. For comfort, Ava compulsively ate. When, as an adult, she got into a twelve-step recovery programme, her father's gifts of money stopped, but his gifts of food continued.

Ava's mother got a companion cat. Perhaps the green eyes of the cat mirrored the envy and hate of Ava's mother because Ava felt terrified of that cat. Seeing Ava's terror, her mother kept the cat in the kitchen or living room whenever she wanted Ava to remain in her room. On those days Ava could not cook or clean. Sometimes she did not attend school because the cat waited outside her door. Ava felt convinced the cat would attack, unsheathe its claws and maul her face. The more frightened she became, the more her mother laughed.

In the first years of our process together, Ava bought her own home, lost the weight she was trying to lose and was awarded a prestigious financially remunerative honour over thousands of other nurses in the hospital where she worked. But then Ava became flooded by an inner certainty that she had trespassed in some way. She had achieved what other nurses had not, what her mother had not. All eyes were on her. It felt to Ava as if she had violated a rule, the rule that she existed to serve others, to help others, and could not triumph in such a visible way. Envy attacks by other nurses reinforced Ava's terror, a terror that quickly became a rage, often directed at me.

'You white people will kill us,' she yelled. And if I tried to explore her statement with something as simple as, 'You sound angry with me,' she yelled louder, saying that I took what she said far too personally, that all white people took things too personally. Didn't I see this was not about me?

While I knew Ava's rage was about her and her mother, about daring visibility and rejection, and I knew her rage was connected to a history of injustice that was much larger than either one of us, I was the person in the room, the white person Ava yelled at. I often felt speechless with my own rage, as if our analytical third became a pure rage.

The analytic third is a way to conceptualize how neither Ava nor I exist as separate psychological entities in the clinical hour. Like mother and infant, our individualities and inter-subjectivities entwine, shape, and create each other. This follows Green's (1975) 'analytic object' and Ogden's (1994) view that the third is formed in the clinical setting, asymmetrically, privileging the unconscious of the patient (ibid).

Rage devoured the connection between Ava and I. Rage thinly veiled our mutual terror of destruction. My mind went numb again and again. When I could sluggishly think, I wondered: Was Ava terrifyingly close to her experience as a child? Was this a forbidden oedipal triumph? Were the intergenerational traumas of slavery and invisibility rising up to shake her from within?

Ava said she drove over to the white area of town to mail letters and buy groceries because the post offices and stores were better. Cleaner. She said a white patient at work called security because she was black and did not do as he asked. He was not even her patient, just saw her in the hall and thought she should roll him over in his bed. 'Your people are something else,' Ava said. She told me black patients were rushed out of the hospital even if they had high blood pressure or other health risks, while white patients were treated with more care. 'Nothing to do about it,' Ava said. 'Your people are trying to kill us off.'

At times I felt defensive, responsible by the colour of my skin, a defensiveness Ava saw and struck at. 'Do you have bars on your windows?' she asked one time. 'In my area of town, we all have bars. If we didn't, we'd be robbed for sure.' And much in the same factual manner, I answered Ava's questions about Christianity, I told her she had the money to buy a house in my neighbourhood, that black people and Latinos and Asians all lived there.

'I have to be with my people,' Ava said.

The psychological legacies of slavery, colonisation, and empire haunt those of us in the United States. Ron Eyerman (2001) refers to the collective experience of African Americans as 'cultural trauma', a term capturing its historical and violent roots. And Farhad Dalal (2006) challenges the more common psychological approach to racism in which 'political rage is understood as a displacement of the "real" internal and personal rage.' Dalal expands psychoanalytic explanations to wonder, 'It is at the very least curious that the self-loathing is *only* understood as a defence, and not as a symptom of living in a racist context' (2006, p. 17, *italics* in original).

I felt more and more helpless as Ava began to self-destruct. She ate compulsively, gaining back sixty pounds she had lost. She married a man she barely knew, an unemployed preacher. He wrecked a car she bought him. Two cars. Three. He had affairs, one with her sister-in-law. Then he began to harm her physically, threatening to burn her house, turning the wheel of her car into oncoming traffic as he drove her to work. Worried about her survival, I suggested marriage therapy. He did not attend the sessions. I suggested divorce, and we argued. 'What about all the other divorced people in your church,' I said. 'They're black. Are they going to hell? Your mother wasn't strong enough to leave. You are'. To which Ava replied: 'You white people all get divorced too easily. You want us black people to be like you. My mother stayed with my father and I can't be better than her. Besides, the Bible doesn't allow divorce'.

Ava and I meet dogs and a cat

Seven years after her marriage, Ava got her divorce. A year after her divorce and thirteen years into our process together, I built out an office at the back of my house, leaving the midrise where I had worked. The rain slowed construction and the walk to my office was incomplete, little more than a trail of mud over which I arranged wood planks. Half an hour into Ava's session, I found her in her car, shaking. She pointed to the mud puddles and planks, screaming, tears running down her face.

You didn't think I would walk up that! You don't know me – you couldn't think that! I went up that other walk, the finished one, and you left your house door unlocked. You white people all leave your doors unlocked and you have so many dogs. You white people will hurt someone with your dogs. You white people in your white neighbourhoods have no idea how people live. You will kill us.

Did the planks over the walk to my office symbolise intergenerational traumas of slaves who walked on planks to care for rice in the region? Did my dogs raise traumatic memories of black people who were hunted by dogs? Perhaps my office door at the back of the house touched the way black people were only allowed access to white people's houses through back doors? Or was an office in my home too close, too personal for Ava? But I could ask no questions because Ava stopped coming to sessions and returned no calls. I felt helpless. Distraught.

In *Ritual and Spontaneity in the Psychoanalytic Process* (1998), Irwin Hoffman explores tensions between an analyst's feeling of connection to patients and the training and expertise. For Hoffman, these tensions cannot be resolved, but are to be attended to through dynamics of psychoanalytic ritual and personal participation.

> To the extent that the analyst conceives of himself or herself merely as offering a service based upon technical expertise, doing analysis can be a relatively comfortable way to make a living. To the extent, however, that the analyst conceives of his or her role, correctly in my view, as combining technical expertise with a special quality of love and affirmation, one that derives part of its power from the inheritance of the mantel of clerical authority, the occupation can be a source of some unspoken and usually disclaimed embarrassment (p. xix).

I felt I had failed Ava. Whatever else had occurred, when she met my dogs, she experienced violation. Animals provided tenderness in the harsh environment of my own childhood, and it did not occur to me she would walk into the midst of my dogs and they would frighten her.

Richard Tan's writing on *Racism and Similarity* (1993) outlines ways both therapist and patient can hide from issues of difference, in particular racial difference, by taking refuge in similarities. This entrenches the dyad in a paranoid-schizoid manner because they become hidden and disassociated from themselves as well as one another. And from the start, Ava and I appeared to enter this dynamic, disassociating our differences in an effort to connect. I often thought of the two of us as sisters in the transference/countertransference: born the same year, both in helping professions, our roots in Christianity, she eating too much in stress and I eating too little, she giving generously and myself more a miser. And in spite of rage erupting into consciousness, by the time Ava met my dogs, I had become so heavily committed to minimizing our differences, I did not create a frame within which she felt safe enough to risk.

After six long months, Ava reconnected. She had just assaulted a co-worker. 'Management made me go to a therapist for anger', she said. 'That one cost less money and I wanted her to work, but she said things I already know'.

In the interim, in addition to the four rescue dogs Ava bumped into inside my house, I had adopted a local family of feral cats. One of the cats became ill, so I kept it in my back office for recovery, away from the consulting room. The cat lay quiet for weeks but then began to use the curtain as a lever to lift the door, push it open and enter the consulting room. Remembering Ava's fear of cats, and her terror when meeting my dogs – no longer blinded by a haze of similarity – I locked the cat into the bathroom for Ava's sessions, where the door could be dead-bolted. Ava refused to enter the office until the cat was locked away. 'You know, if that cat gets loose, I will leave and never come back,' she said. Scratches covered my arms from restraining the cat. I wrote signs on the bathroom door: Closed for Cat. I hired a contractor and got a new deadbolt for the back office so the cat could no longer use the curtain as a lever.

Ava spoke of the cat every session: that it was my cat and I locked it behind a door. She began to calm down, bringing in a video of two children playing with a muddy puppy in a bathtub, crying as she played it for me: 'It's like a baby. I never knew pets were so much like children'. And although Ava still spoke of race, it was no longer as angrily. Rather, she explained her culture and experience, trying to help me understand. She began to lose the weight she had gained and changed her home church to one with women pastors as well as men. 'The Prozac I've taken all these years must finally be working', Ava said and smiled. 'I even have compassion for your animal craziness'.

And when I asked about using our work together in papers I write, Ava told me she would be honoured if her struggle could be of use to others. Yet I felt uncomfortable, wondering if I once again entered some enactment of similarity. I asked again. She agreed again. I asked a third time, and Ava became angry: 'No, girlfriend. You have your writing and your animal craziness. That's you, girlfriend. It's not me. And you keep asking me the same question over and over. That's your issue, not mine.'

A cat as part of the frame

There is great anxiety deconstructing familiar narratives. The race is a familiar narrative. When Ava chose to work with me, she demonstrated her willingness to engage difference and race, issues that cannot easily be separated from dynamics of early maternal attachment as cultural, family, and gender expectations are absorbed with the gleam in our parents' eyes.

Harriet Kimble Wrye and Judith K. Welles explore these dynamics in *The Narration of Desire: Erotic Transferences and Countertransferences* (1994). For Wrye and Welles, pre-oedipal, nonverbal issues are often brought into treatment in the form of representative objects of the patient's body. Such objects are symbolic of a defect felt by the patient, a defect felt to be present from the earliest history (ibid). The concrete quality of these enactments feels necessary to the patients because words cannot adequately convey the experience:

> Typically the patient was unable to carry on in the analytic mode, was unable to talk about feeling, and felt compelled instead to action. Something primitive, preverbal and maybe even terrible was going on (Wrye and Welles, 1994, p. 22).

Work with Ava was filled with concrete transference/countertransference enactments, from our first discussion of Christianity and my mind's pattern of shutting down, to her bringing me clothes catalogues so I would 'dress better', and spilling chocolate chip ice cream in the waiting room. Ava struggled to verbalize her sense of defect in a way I could understand.

Carl Jung (Jung and Baynes, 1921) understood any true symbol to be the best possible description of a relatively unknown fact. That is, by the time a symbol is fully captured in words, fully made conscious and known, it no longer operates as a symbol that bridges the conscious and unconscious, because it exists primarily in the realm of conscious knowledge (ibid). Such a view brings into question the primacy of words, a precursor to the relational school's work on enactments when a mix of transference/countertransference is acted into without conscious awareness. As Donnel Stern says, 'enacted experience is unformulated experience' (2004, p. 212). Much like Jung's view of the symbol, within the enactment are myriad hints or possibilities as to what it means, where it comes from, what it is about. And by the time the enacted experience is formed into an accessible, useful interpretation, it is no longer filled with as much raw potential or unconscious dread.

Whatever else it was, the symbol/enactment of the cat I restrained during the clinical hour became much more than a cat for both Ava and me. The cat's tiny mewing and soft weight of its body echoed the sounds and feel of an infant, connecting it to pre-oedipal issues – messy, demanding instincts that raged, hungered, desired. In addition, Ava's mother had once used a cat as an extension of herself to torture Ava. The cat symbolized division. Alienation. The cat symbolized hate. Wrye and Welles (1994) observe that 'patients who are most terrified of experiencing primitive body sensation and longing associate them to a loss of control' (p. 105). In this way, the cat symbolized restraint, my restraining of myself – my rage and desire to merge – and by transference extension, Ava's mother's restraint. The cat came to represent both the Winnicottian version of hate (1986), which developmentally based hate the child learns to recognize as coexisting with love, and a bridge through the cultural hatreds of racism filled with malevolence and violence. But perhaps most significantly, the cat symbolized my capacity to keep Ava in mind as different from myself. I could prepare a ritual frame for our clinical hour together where inside and outside were separate enough for Ava to risk vulnerability and self-reflection, to find her own meaning.

There is no longer an easy division between words and actions in the clinical hour. The choice to speak or not speak is as much an action as my choice to lock up the cat. I will never fully know what the cat has meant to Ava, but it has served as a link between us, and with that link are new/old questions.

In the story told by the Sufi masters, the cat was once restrained because it disrupted meditation. Then the community memory eclipsed the purpose of restraining the cat. The ritual became hollowed out. Empty.

It seems to me that those of us engaged in the work of psychoanalysis and psychotherapy are often at the brink of such hollow rituals. To understand that restraining the cat was of use to Ava is one thing but believing that restraining the cat will continue to be of use to Ava is quite another, and no less damaging than my desire to ignore our differences and focus on similarity.

References

Dalal, F. (2006) Racism: Processes of detachment, dehumanization, and hatred. In K. White (ed.),*Unmasking Race, Culture, and Attachment in the Psychoanalytic Space*. Karnac: London, pp. 10–35.

Eyerman, R. (2001) *Cultural Trauma: Slavery and the Formation of African American Identity*. Cambridge: Cambridge University Press.

Green, A. (1975) The analyst, symbolization and absence in the analytic setting. *International Journal of Psychoanalysis*, 56(1), pp. 1–22.

Hoffman, I.Z. (1998) *Ritual and Spontaneity in the Psychoanalytic Process: A Dialectical-Constructivist View*. London: Analytic Press.

Jung, C.G. and Baynes, H.G. (1921) *Psychological Types; Collected Works*, Volume 6. London: Routledge.

Mitchell, S.A. (1993) *Hope and Dread in Psychoanalysis*. New York: Basic Books.

Ogden, T. (1994) *Subjects of Analysis*. London: Jason Aronson Inc.

Shah, I. (1988) *The Magic Monastery: Analogical and Action Philosophy of the Middle East and Central Asia*. London: ISF.

Stern, D.B. (2004) The eye sees itself: Dissociation, enactment, and the achievement of conflict. *Contemporary Psychoanalysis*, 40(2), pp. 197–237.

Tan, R. (1993) Racism and similarity: Paranoid-schizoid structures. *British Journal of Psychotherapy,* 10(1), pp. 33–43.

Winnicott, D.W. (1986) *Home is Where We Start From: Essays by a Psychoanalyst*. London: Analytic Press.

Wrye, H.K. and Welles, J. (1994) *The Narration of Desire: Erotic Transference and Countertransference*. London: Analytic Press.

12 Like a bridge over troubled waters

Beth Feldman

Introduction

I sit across from our patient with my carefully chosen words. He sits next to our patient with raw, drooling emotion. I sit back in my chair with crossed legs, the epitome of personal boundaries and social convention. He lays on his back, paws up – the embodiment of childlike trust and innocence.

The relational magic that a dog brings to the psychoanalytic consulting room has a unique influence on the quality of the analytic relationship – a relationship which underlies the analyst's ability to bring about intrapsychic change and interpersonal healing. A dog in the consulting room can function like a bridge over troubled waters, helping patients and analysts reach the unconscious and dissociated and helping them reach each other. As the unabashedly needy dog, often complete with his own history of early trauma, warms the analytic space, he elicits feelings of acceptance and belonging that relax the chains of emotional guardedness and encourage more spontaneous and authentic relatedness. Case examples will demonstrate how this furry creature functions as a third in the treatment room, infusing the air with currents of primal need and basic trust and eliciting preoedipal and oedipal longings. The dog as a magnet for projections, identifications and dissociated self-states, as well as an emotional barometer for many patients, will be examined as well via case examples.

The relational magic of the dog

What enables a person to share her deepest shame, to experience and give voice to feelings that she has had to tuck away in the attic of her being? What gives someone the courage to put aside a lifetime of feeling misunderstood and test the waters of emotional closeness? What is the 'unleashing' influence of a dog in the room on the psychoanalytic process? For me, the answer to these questions involves the unique quality of the analytic relationship and how this relationship lives in the analytic space, both of which are influenced by the presence of my dog in the room. I have considered what helps me to be my most emotionally available, authentic self with my patients and what creates an analytic space which encourages this unique kind of relationship to take hold and flourish? With these concerns in mind, I have a bright red leather chair in my office for an infusion of vitality, gold and brown sconces on the wall for the warm glow of filtered light and a candle burning in the corner for the relaxation that the sight and the scent of the single flame evokes. Most importantly, I add a dog to the room for the unspoken promise of relational magic that dogs so often bring.

As I began my analytic training several years ago, I informed my supervisor that I often had one of my dogs in sessions with me. 'Who is he there for' she asked, 'your patients or you?' 'Both' was the answer I eventually was able to offer. I was beginning to understand how this extra body in the room could be instrumental as an agent of change for my patients and greatly facilitated my work as an analyst.

Dogs have always had a central place in my emotional world. They exert a gravitational pull that has made me feel loved and balanced throughout my life. Dogs warm the air that I breathe and relax the bones of my conscious mind, allowing thought, emotion and words to flow more freely. Interacting in the presence of people can be like navigating a busy street for me, filled with instructions, prohibitions and rules that taunt my contrary nature. Interacting in the presence of a dog feels like a beach in the early morning – open, with endless possibilities and hints of promised joy. As an analyst, my dog's centering, calming presence helps me be more relaxed, focused and emotionally present with my patients.

My first dog, Jenny, was my best friend throughout my childhood and adolescent years. She offered the unconditional love and acceptance that I didn't always find in the two-legged world, as well as companionship and an adventurous spirit that I grew to rely upon. The summer before my senior year of college and a year after Jenny passed away, I got my own dog. It was Winston, my very feisty Welsh Terrier who helped me select a husband, survive graduate school and taught me about the value of a dog as a co-therapist.

I began including a dog in my pre-graduate schoolwork as a crisis counselor at a residential facility for adolescent girls. Winston and I worked twenty-four-hour shifts in the crisis house where I was called to intervene when a resident's behavior was out of control. I was tasked with calming or 'physically managing' the upset teen and then somehow, bringing her to the crisis house where Winston and I were the only staff.

Truth be told, I was terrified of more than a few of these girls. Winston was my ambassador, always walking into the room first, disarming the battle-ready teenager with his wet nose and wagging tail. I saw how he relaxed them and how I gained credibility in the adolescent world by being his second in command.

Years later, with a Ph.D. in hand, I set up a pet therapy program at the Children's Day Hospital where I was working. These behaviorally challenged, oppositional children would work their behavior modification programs and achieve impressive levels of behavioral compliance to earn group time with the therapy dogs. The most aggressive children were calm, even tender with the dogs and often briefly, with the staff as well.

As a seasoned clinician in private practice, my dog Justin is frequently in session with me. Justin is a seven-year-old, brown and white poodle mix with bright hazel eyes and floppy ears. He typically greets each patient as they walk in and, if encouraged, will sit with them for much of the session. Justin's presence influences the analytic space and the analytic relationship in a myriad of ways, as I'll demonstrate late on. He offers an infusion of warmth and a hint of spontaneity, and is both a magnet for patients' projections and identifications and an emotional barometer in the treatment room. An extension of me and an object of my love and care, Justin becomes a third in the room, stirring old longings and conflicts and intensifying the transference. Justin wields a subtle but important influence on my internal experience in the room as well.

Having Justin in the room slows time down for me by the slightest measure. As my pace slows, silences can incubate, words can linger, and feelings can fill the air in a less hurried way. I tend to feel more relaxed in his presence and better able to stay emotionally present in the room. My nonverbal ability to connect and resonate with my dogs is channeled in the consulting room. The calming influence of Justin's presence helps me to stay open to the nonverbal, often to what both my patients and I are not allowing ourselves to feel, never mind put into words. This sensitivity for the unarticulated and the dissociated that my relationship with dogs has helped me hone has been instrumental in my gaining a deeper, fuller understanding of my patients and the unique selves that live within them.

Having a dog in the treatment room has not been without its conflicts for me. While I find the presence of my dog in the room to be personally soothing, some patients find Justin to be a distraction, even an annoyance. In such cases, my attention may be divided, concerned that Justin may meander over and pay unwanted attention to a patient. Some have felt that Justin's presence is evidence that, like the narcissistic mother of their childhood, I prioritize my own needs at their expense. He is felt to take away from my ability to focus on them rather than to facilitate it. I have, in fact, found myself distracted by Justin's occasional scratching or roaming or by his unique reaction to certain patients.

Sometimes, Justin has wanted to sit with me when clearly, he could better serve the analytic moment by sitting with my patient. If I let Justin sit with me, I risk becoming the self-serving mother, addressing my own needs while I leave my child hungry and wanting. If I give Justin cues to stay down, I may become the cold and dismissive mother, as they identify with Justin's rejection as the needy, annoying child. At the very least, a dog in the treatment room is a draw for my attention and inevitably adds a dimension of unpredictability within the analytic space which may not always be in the service of the patient's agenda.

Finally, with the presence of a furry other in the analytic space, both the room and I become profoundly less 'blank'. I am a person who has a dog and chooses to bring this dog to work. Just as my wedding ring offers personal data and my casual style of dress and penchant for bright colors suggests other qualities, my wish/need to bring my dog to work may spark questions about my emotional makeup. Am I one of those 'crazy therapists' saddled by my own anxiety disorder or barely contained eccentricity? Do I struggle with a rebellious nature or a narcissistic preoccupation in which my desire to have my dog with me trumps my patients' needs and desires? Or, does the dog's presence suggest to patients that I share with them basic needs for closeness, comfort and connection that feels more accessible in the presence of a dog?

The relational magic of the dog feels related to the sense of comfort and belonging that they generate, facilitating the risking of trust and closeness between patient and analyst. The dog's presence in the treatment room can stir needs and longings that are often fiercely guarded against in human interactions. Justin's reactions are not shackled by human defenses or preconceptions about what is appropriate and therapeutic. Rather, as his presence seems to exude a sense of unconditional acceptance, a mutuality organically emerges between him and those with whom he engages. As the dog comforts and relaxes a patient, previously avoided or dissociated feelings such as longings for closeness, rivalry, envy and rage may be stimulated and left very alive in the analytic space.

I'm with him: the dog's influence on the development of the early therapeutic relationship

The influence of the dog in the room can first be felt in how his presence affects a patient's initial comfort with me and the decision to pursue treatment. Josh's parents sat nervously in my office during our initial consultation. His father spoke in a slow, controlled manner and told me that it was possible that his fifteen-year-old son had an eating disorder. Furthermore, he went on, it was possible that Josh had questions about his sexuality. Josh's mother sat quietly, head down as her husband spoke, stroking Justin methodically with both hands as he sat on the couch next to her. She said little throughout the session but when I asked her if she had any questions, she responded, 'No, you will be fine. You're a member of the tribe'.

'The tribe?', I asked, sure that she was referring to her assumption that I was Jewish, as were they. 'A dog person' she clarified and then added 'Josh will be able to talk to you.' And so, one of the most memorable treatments of my career began. Over the next few years, Josh's parents struggled in and out of sessions to understand their son's very serious bulimia, his bisexuality and his need for antidepressant medication to combat significant feelings of depression. Throughout my work with Josh and at times his parents, Justin was there as a quiet presence who breathed comfort into the room and reassured them that as members of the same tribe, I would understand and not judge them.

The feelings of warmth, acceptance and comfort that many patients describe in the presence of a dog are certainly not universal. One young woman comes to mind who walked by Justin with barely a glance during her first session, announcing smugly that she is a cat person. Not surprisingly, she did not come back for a second session. I too felt the match was not a good one and felt some measure of relief that I would not be tasked with bridging this interpersonal divide.

Working with a dog in my office seems to have a more conscious and apparent influence on my work in the initial, rapport building phase with teenagers than with adults. Having a dog work with me seems to suggest to adolescents that I might be an adult with a small 'a' rather than with a capital 'A'. For many teens, dogs connote trust, acceptance, spontaneity and warmth; antidotes to their view of adults as critical and unable to understand their emotional experiences. Certainly, having a playful, comforting figure in a place that feels alien, where they are charged with a frightening task, seems to be a helpful surprise. This surprise often buys me an opportunity to show what kind of adult I am.

Leah is a highly anxious sixteen-year-old girl who has tolerated but eventually rejected three therapists in six years. According to Leah, one just played games with her and 'it was useless'. One talked about herself too much and had Leah's mother in the room half the time. The third therapist didn't speak enough, appeared too formal and seemed to be put off by Leah's edgy 'adults suck' attitude.

Leah's mother warned me in our initial consultation that their relationship was quite strained and that her daughter saw therapy as her mother's ploy to better control her behavior. I had the sense that I would come to agree with Leah on this one and began to resonate with her wish to rebel against her mother's efforts to use her as a means to quell her own anxieties.

When Leah entered the office for her first session, I introduced myself and then the poodle who was excitedly wagging his tail at her feet. She fell to her knees to greet Justin with equal enthusiasm, abandoning her armor of adolescent indifference. I quickly fell within the shadow of the instant connection Leah felt toward Justin and was deemed worthy of a chance.

Leah spoke at length about her highly conflictual relationship with her intrusive and controlling mother who, Leah was certain, preferred her younger brother. She professed indifference to this but quickly agreed that her constant anger toward her mother might suggest that this was painful to her. Leah described lifelong struggles with anxiety, sadness and an exquisite sensitivity to separation. Throughout this very powerful first session, Leah sat with Justin on her lap. She stroked his shoulders with both hands, a gesture that served to both soothe her and help her pace herself.

For Leah, like many adolescents, the dog was felt to be a good object, understanding and accepting. Adults represented the promise of being many kinds of objects; the nurturing and holding mother, the anxious and intrusive mother, the critical and rejecting mother to name a few. Relationships with adults raise the likelihood of bumping into a combination of these internal mothers and as such, are both longed for and fiercely guarded against. Justin, on the other hand, sits by them as they rant, cry or shut down; a quiet, comforting object who reaffirms that they are lovable and not alone.

For most patients who have sought treatment with me, Justin's presence has been a welcome surprise. While each patient forms his own relationship with him, most respond to Justin's warmth and affection, experiencing it as a welcome balance to my analytic reserve. They appear touched by his enthusiasm at seeing them as he wags his tail excitedly and follows them from the door to the couch. They can hold him, pet him and often receive the comfort of a cold nose sniffing them should they appear visibly upset. He notices, he cares and he acts – in sharp contrast to my often ineffectual world of words.

The dog as a third in the treatment room: eliciting pre-oedipal and oedipal longings

A dog in the consulting room can transform the analytic space in ways which facilitate the deepening of the analytic relationship. The dog can become a third (Benjamin, 2012) in the room, functioning as a bridge from the unconscious to the conscious and from the intrapsychic to the interpersonal, stirring longings from childhood that might remain more difficult to access within the strictly two-person analyst/patient dynamic. As wishes for the merger, issues around separation and individuation and feelings of competition come alive with the dog's emergence as a third, they become available for processing and integration.

Freud (1920) focused on the concept of the third in the parents/child relationship, as he placed the oedipal triangle in the center of a young child's psychosexual development and a central theme revived in transference configurations. Issues related to rivalry, competition and aggression are stirred by the oedipal dynamics and feelings of arousal/rejection and specialness/exclusion may emerge as connected to primal scene issues. Freud considered oedipal issues, i.e. developmental challenges related to the child being the third with his mother and father, to be important for healthy psychosexual and emotional development and successful adult functioning. It is worth noting that Freud often had a dog with him during sessions.

More recently, Thomas Ogden (2004) suggested that the construction of the analytic third is a function of the subjectivity of both the patient and the analyst. While the patient's subjectivity is the focus of concern and inquiry, the analyst's examination of her experience in and of the analytic third is used as a bridge to understanding the internal world of the patient. In his discussion of the creation and influence of the analytic third, Ogden writes, 'experiences in and of the analytic third often generate a quality of intimacy between patient and analyst [and] these experiences in the analytic third may hold particular importance to the analysis in that they may be the first instances in the patient's life of such healthy, generative forms of object re-lationships' (Ogden, 2004, p. 237).

Jessica Benjamin (2012) speaks about the third as the potential relational knowing that can emerge and inhabit the psychoanalytic space in the room and in the analytic relationship, such that each can temporarily surrender their own view and consider the view of the separate other. Given the dog's widespread experience as an object which offers unconditional love and ac-ceptance, one could suggest that this generates a sense of interpersonal rec-ognition and knowing in the other. Might both patient and analyst project their need to feel seen and known onto the dog, utilizing the furry other as a third in the psychoanalytic space? While relational theorists have focused on the creation of an analytic third in the analytic encounter, this chapter explores how the physical presence of a third, in this case a dog, may act as a repository for projections from both participants' subjectivities.

The nature of the dog's embodiment of the analytic third is, in part de-pendent on the developmental needs of the patient. Some patients struggling with pre-oedipal concerns use Justin as an extension of me and as such, as an object with which to merge. Others use Justin as a transitional object of sorts, merging with him while making early attempts at tolerating sep-aration from me. This has often been the case when patients make early, anxiety-laden attempts at expressing anger at me.

Patients with more primitive ego development are often not able to toler-ate even a whiff of separation. The presence of Justin as a third may inter-fere with their symbiotic transference needs. Such patients have an inability to tolerate experiencing the analyst as a separate whole object, with her own needs, experiences and especially with her own 'other'. As living proof of the analyst's separateness and therefore the patient's aloneness, the dog puts the patient at risk of being exposed as vulnerable and unformed, a fledgling chick, unable to fend for himself and unable to fly away. The presence of a dog in the treatment room may be difficult for these patients as feelings of envy, rage and a need to destroy the good object to which they don't feel they have sufficient access, may dominate their experience (Segal, 1964).

My work with Warren, a severely depressed, highly intellectualized and obsessional forty-year-old man offers an example of a patient with debilitat-ing pre-oedipal struggles and of how having a dog in the room influenced our work together. I treated Warren in two times weekly psychoanalytic treatment for seven years. Warren sought analysis to help him manage over-whelming feelings of depression and crippling panic attacks. As the oldest of three boys, Warren described the feeling that he was never smart enough, popular enough or handsome enough for either his vain, narcissistic mother or extremely intellectual and emotionally limited father. He was particularly self-conscious about his height, as he stands five feet, six inches tall. Our relationship was marked by his need to demean me as paid help who was obligated to listen to the obsessional details of his life. He would deliver his longwinded monologues with a painfully monotonous tone and become enraged at any attempt on my part to interrupt with a question, clarification or even an empathic response. As with the prostitutes he hires, I was expected to meet his needs, absorb his rage and have no feelings or needs of my own, especially as he routinely let me know how unhelpful I was and what a disappointment I had become to him.

Justin was experienced by Warren as an intruder and a rival, the favored baby while he was the despised and burdensome oldest child. As such, Justin was the 'other' that stood in the way of his merger with me and triggered a rage that helped fuel his weekly destruction of me. Warren would glare at Justin with disdain as the dog lay equidistant between us on my office rug. He was focused on my quickest glance in Justin's direction and would become enraged if my attention splintered for even a second.

Warren was quick to comment that I wasn't giving him my full attention and he wasn't paying me to look at my dog. We talked about what it meant to him that I had something, someone of my own in the session with me. This led to an outpouring of rage toward his mother, as he described how his hyperactivity and poor social skills left him in a near-constant state of being criticized by his rejecting, self-centered mother. He also talked about his disdain for his brothers, both of whom he felt got the love and encouragement that he was denied.

Thus, as feelings of envy and jealousy emerged toward Justin, we were able to gingerly reflect on Warren's internal experience growing up in a family where he felt despised and emotionally abandoned. His hatred toward me as the self-involved mother of his childhood was facilitated by Justin's presence in the room.

Unlike most patients, Warren never spoke to Justin or allowed himself to receive any of the warmth and affection that Justin would offer. As the favored child, Justin was the recipient of Warren's disdain, usually manifested in his frequent scowling at the dog and complaints about his presence. After seven years of twice a week treatment, I can remember suddenly having the fantasy in the middle of a session, that Warren was going to viciously kick Justin. Several weeks later, he precipitously ended what had been a long and difficult treatment for both of us, by unleashing a series of highly aggressive, threatening voicemails, declaring that he was firing me. While I will never know exactly what the guilty match was that torched our treatment, my separateness as evidenced by my having an 'other' in the room, was undoubtedly part of his torment.

Justin served the vital function of keeping me alive in my sessions with Warren. His suffocating need to consume me, to focus on my every move, always attributing petty or self-serving motives to my offerings, was barely tolerable as a steady diet during our twice-weekly sessions. The depth of his loathing of me, of himself and of the few others in his small world, was toxic. Perhaps most of all, his inability to let me join him in any way was deadening and left survival as the only goal for all three of us.

For me, Justin's presence felt like an island of good in a sea of bad objects that flooded the treatment room. When I felt erased by his dissociated, obsessive soliloquies or overwhelmed by his venomous verbal assaults, Justin was a centering force whose presence helped me keep my analytic footing through the worst of Warren's storms.

For Ava, a thirty-five-year-old young woman with anxiety and depression, Justin was the preferred sibling but unlike Warren, she could tolerate the intrusion between us and the rivalrous feelings that emerged. Ava desperately wanted more closeness and nurturance from me and experienced the limits of the therapeutic relationship as an indication that I didn't care about her. She seemed to wish that like Justin, she could curl up in my lap, be scratched behind the ear and be taken home at the end of the day. Ava alternated between patting Justin and talking to him as he sat by her side and questioning how I would feel about her if she didn't like dogs or complained about his presence in the session. This led us to talk about how hard it was for her as a child to ask directly to have her needs met or give voice to her anger and resentment lest her barely engaged mother detach completely.

Early anxiety around attachment has made authentic relatedness very difficult for Ava. Her overwhelming wish for closeness and experience of boundaries and limits as rejection precluded engaging in age-appropriate competition with her younger siblings. Ava resorted to splitting off many of the more challenging, impressive facets of her personality in favor of the superficial, people-pleasing persona which was congruent with the role assigned to her within her family. Ava used her relationship with Justin as both a way to seek approval and closeness from me and as a way to test out my responsiveness to her anger and fledgling self-assertiveness. Must she continue to be, like Justin, and her longstanding role within her family, there to meet the needs and fulfill the expectations of others? By both identifying with Justin and competing with him, Ava was learning to give voice to her sadness and anger and pay attention to her own very impressive intellect.

For Ava, Justin has significant transference implications. Ava has struggled throughout her thirty-five years to get the warmth, attention and nurturance that she needed from her very reserved, intellectual mother. Her reactions to Justin and what emerged between the three of us brought core interpersonal issues to the forefront for Ava.

Ava studied my interactions with Justin during sessions. Was I the loving, longed-for mother with Justin, holding him and comforting him as we talked? Did I ignore Justin and in doing so, become the emotionally distant mother of her childhood? She would often muse about the kind of mother she thinks I am, identifying with Justin's longing and seeing me, much like her own mother, as cold and withholding. More recently, Ava has been able to experience me as more loving and actively struggles with the sadness and anger that the tender nurturance that she has always longed for routinely went to a younger, in her eyes, preferred sibling.

Justin's presence in the room seems to have facilitated Ava's experience of a negative maternal transference that has allowed her to experience an angry, ignored, emotionally starved self-state, an internal experience that she has fought to sequester since she was a young child. By stimulating early needs and sibling issues, Justin facilitated the unfolding of a rageful part of herself that she has sacrificed in the service of staying close to important others in her life. Simultaneously, he provided warmth and comfort and represented a connection to me that allowed Ava to tolerate these terribly uncomfortable feelings.

In my work with Ava, Justin served as a bridge for me to gain access certain split off parts of myself. Justin helped me travel in sessions back to my own rivalrous experience with preferred siblings. In his relaxed, soothing presence, I could identify with her split off rage and understand the price exacted in terms of ego development, that this ongoing accommodation has cost her. Not only did she abort the development of her very keen intellect, she painstakingly cultivated a beautiful shell that encased a self with troublesome pockets of emptiness. Ava's bubbly, people-pleasing persona was her interpersonal offering that was always at the expense of feeling truly known and authentically connected to the other. Thus, as Justin helped me gain access in sessions to the underbelly of my own attempts to cope, he helped me connect with what was split off and sacrificed by Ava.

The dog as a third invites spontaneity

The dog's unscripted presence in the analytic space suggests that spontaneity and unpredictability are welcome. Dogs bring movement to the room and hint that we do not need to stay locked in the traditional world of words. While the therapeutic experience is traditionally a verbal one, spontaneous action can break through what may feel like impenetrable resistance, a sense of deadness or intractable symptoms.

The focus on the potential mutative impact of the dog's unpredictability in the treatment room is supported by the work of the Boston Change Process Study Group. The Boston Change Process Study Group (2005) looked at the process of change in psychotherapy and focused on the nuances of the moment to moment interactions between patient and therapist. They talked about noninterpretive factors, the 'something more' that brings about change in the therapeutic process and focused on an indeterminate 'fuzziness', 'sloppiness' and 'unpredictability' (p. 693) as being instrumental in clinical change.

My work with Dee, a painfully depressed and extremely isolated twenty-two-year-old woman exemplifies how spontaneity, fostered by the presence of a dog in the room, filled the analytic space and rescued a stagnating treatment. After two years at a residential treatment facility following many years of school refusal, Dee was severely depressed and rarely left her home. The sick parent she sacrificed her adolescent years to care for, had passed away. Now, the smallest of tasks felt unmanageable and day and night were interchangeable. While Dee's connection with me was strong, her ability to work in the treatment ebbed and flowed, as her depression and anxiety fluctuated from moderate to severe.

One particular session stands out in my mind when Dee uncharacteristically would not make eye contact and muttered under her breath rather than spoke to me. We sat in what felt like a toxic silence for many minutes, a silence which felt like it was smothering the last tendrils of hope in the room. Finally, feeling somewhat lost, I reflected that Dee seemed to be in a darker place than I had seen her in a long time. After another long silence, I said, 'That's ok, I'll just rest there with you'. We sat quietly for what again felt like an eternity. Searching for my footing in this depressive abyss, I mused about the dark area in what I shared was my favorite picture in my office. I told her that this area looked like isolated, distant mountains to me and made me think of the part of her that felt so far away and terribly alone. Dee spoke quietly, still not looking at me and said that those were not mountains but rather, they were rocks with the ocean's waves crashing all around them. I leapt out of my chair and examined the picture in question up close. Within a second, Dee and Justin were up too, and Dee was pointing out where she saw the rocks and the water. She acknowledged that she could see how I might see them as mountains, but she maintained her view that it was waves crashing around the rocks. There was eye contact. There was animation in our voices. There was affect in the air. There was life. A month later, Dee enrolled in community college, and a month after that, she began classes.

I am not suggesting that Justin was responsible for this surprise moment in Dee's treatment. While he did not lead the charge toward the painting, his uninhibited, action-oriented way of being in the room made both my jumping up and Dee's jumping up, feel less out of place. The three of us created this moment which fused movement with the unchaining of Dee's self-imposed isolation.

The dog as a barometer in the treatment room

Justin influences the analytic space by acting as an emotional barometer for my patients, helping them experience, appreciate and manage the intensity of their affect. While I do my level best not to fall out of my chair or appear rattled when a patient begins to rage at me, Justin feels no such need for this limitation. He might look up in a startling way or jump down from their side in response to unusual yelling. Often when a patient would cry or appear visibly upset, he might park himself next to her as a source of comfort, as an affect regulator. My concern initially was that patients would be soothed and quieted, receiving an implicit message that strong affect is discouraged. In fact, however, the opposite seems to happen. Patients seem to feel that they can unleash less comfortable feelings such as anger and deep sadness, with Justin literally by their side.

Philip Bromberg (2008) suggests that fear of emotional dysregulation drives the tendency for dissociation. He focuses on the presence of both safety and risk in the analytic relationship as key factors underlying the mutative impact of the analytic relationship. The dog's ability to enhance feelings of safety in the consulting room for patient and analyst alike seem to result in the patient's feeling contained and accepted such that they are then able to risk experiencing and expressing painful affect.

Alan is a forty-five-year-old man with a long history of substance abuse, tumultuous interpersonal relationships and severe irritability. Alan grew up with an alcoholic father and bore witness to his father beating his mother for the smallest perceived slight. Alan despised himself for his inability to protect his mother, a betrayal made worse by the feelings of love he still felt for his father. As an adult, Alan experiences his father's extreme sensitivity to slights and frustrations and has relied on drugs, high-risk behaviors and physical aggression to manage his rage and feelings of vulnerability.

As Alan became sober and worked in therapy, he began to experience and eventually manage his kaleidoscope of emotions. He is driven by a determination to be 'nothing like that prick' and sees himself as a fierce protector of his mother, sister and girlfriend. Though he works tirelessly in therapy, has daily workouts in the gym and is on antidepressant medication to help with his irritability, Alan is still hobbled by his volatility. What used to be holes punched in the wall or bouts of verbal abuse that cost him past relationships, has been whittled down to an angry raised voice, with clenched teeth and balled fists. Alan is incredulous when his girlfriend complains about his aggressive behavior as he feels he is turning himself inside out to not release his rage. While he challenges his girlfriend's experience of his outbursts as well as my own as threatening, he is moved by Justin's startled reactions to his anger in sessions. He believes that the women in his life overreact to his admitted 'temper' but Justin's jumping off his chair and scurrying halfway across the room is experienced as the gold standard of the truth.

As Alan became able to register the reaction of the 'other' to his rage, he became increasingly able to experience and reflect upon the waxing of irritability into anger and anger into fury. Feelings of shame and helplessness emerged as Alan could see the shadows of his father's rage coming alive within him but seemed easier for Alan to tolerate with Justin's steady presence by his side.

Alan's developing ability to tolerate his rage and connect childhood feelings of powerlessness to his present-day explosions has helped him stay sober, function better in the work world and has transformed his ability to be a partner in his intimate relationship. I believe that Justin's accepting, calming presence in the room was one of the special ingredients that has enabled his growth in our work together.

The bridge

Working as a bridge from the unconscious to the conscious and from the intrapsychic to the interpersonal, the presence of a dog in the analytic space can enhance a sense of safety in the analytic relationship, encouraging the unfolding of progressive communication and unconscious processes. As a magnet for projections and identifications, the dog triggers early memories, wishes, needs and fears. As such, the dog sometimes falls within the shadow of the transference, stirring feelings about the therapist as a parent and feelings of sibling rivalry. The presence of a dog encourages the experience of strong affect and provides a comfort that facilitates the experience of split off affects and self-states. Finally, the dog sometimes is used as a self-object, providing the holding, comforting and mirroring functions that are typically reserved for the two-legged therapist.

Jen, a sixty-five-year-old recovered alcoholic, struggled with severe depression and isolation so profound, it chilled me to the bone. She felt emotionally abandoned by a narcissistic mother who lacked the patience or inclination to focus on Jen's emotional needs. Jen was the youngest of three children and was seen as difficult and demanding by the adults in her world. She focused on her attractiveness as her only source of narcissistic supplies. Jen became an impulsive teenager, with little sense of self and even less ability to self-reflect or self-regulate.

As an adult, Jen could not succeed in a career as a model, was unable to engage in meaningful work and failed in her three significant intimate relationships. She blamed years of substance abuse and depression for the many disappointments and failures in her adult life and exuded a sense that she saw herself as inherently damaged and unredeemable.

Jen seemed torn in treatment, desperately inhaling the contact and interest that was taken in her, while feeling hopeless that anything could temper the depth of her resentment, isolation and self-hate. Jen identified with Justin, responding to him as one unfortunate stray to another. She would pat him while talking and almost seemed to be speaking for the two of them. Jen would talk about feeling that she didn't have a home or a family, just a studio apartment and no one in the world who truly cared about her. She watched a world of people with lives that seemed filled with love and purpose but felt unable to have even crumbs of either in her life.

Jen talked about feelings of helplessness and futility. She felt unable to sustain a relationship, manage her very labile mood or find an interest to fill her many empty hours. Unlike other emotional outcasts, Jen couldn't even find a home in the twelve-step programs. While she held onto a vague, unarticulated hope of being rescued, this hope was made all the more unlikely by her irritability and desperate, off-putting interpersonal style.

Earlier in treatment, Jen identified with Justin as an abandoned stray and talked about feelings of loneliness, rejection and helplessness. As her depression worsened and the transference deepened, Jen related to Justin as the preferred, more lovable sibling who was cherished in a way that she would never experience. Anger and resentment accompanied her desperate sadness, as Jen struggled to stay connected to me and battle the dragons of despair that lived inside her.

During one session, Jen was staring at me silently. After several moments I asked, 'What are you thinking?' 'I'm wishing I was you.' Jen responded with a melancholy voice and piercing stare that left me speechless. As this mixture of despair and envy filled the room, I slowly regained my ability to use words and quietly said, 'Tell me more'. 'Oh, Dr. Feldman' she sighed, with an intensity of feeling, 'to be you. To have a home and a family and a dog and a life. To be you'.

As a good object in her world, Justin embodied the twinning selfobject properties of unconditional acceptance and identification as an abandoned emotional stray. Wolf's (1988) description of the twinship selfobject transference as '[t]he need to experience the essential likeness of the selfobject and to be strengthened by its quietly sustaining presence' (p. 58) highlights one facet of the supportive function that Justin provided. In the end, however, both he and I were inadequate as selfobjects, our tepid offers of caring and concern like the offer of an umbrella in the midst of a tsunami.

As a bad object, Justin became the victor in her world of sibling rivalry, appropriating the lion's share of the maternal attention and affection that she so desperately needed. Both he and I indulged our emotional greed, excluding her from the heart of our world and sharing only forty-five-minute scraps of our lives with her. As such, we gave form to the rage and envy that swirled through her internal world and became key players in Jen's tragic enactment. Seeking revenge against the mothers who would never love her enough and the siblings who lived gluttonous lives of emotional (and financial) plenty, Jen's suicide was her silent scream, 'Look what you made me do!'

In the end, Jen felt condemned to a lifetime of interpersonal homelessness. While I had hoped that Justin and I could offer her something, someone to hold onto, our real-world presence offered far too little, far too late. Depleted by decades of swimming in the muck of profound isolation and despair, Jen ultimately used Justin and myself as the recorders of her tragic history. In the end, she counted on us to be witnesses and the lone souls who might miss her after she took her own life.

Dennis, a thirty-seven-year-old single man entered treatment six years ago seeking help for a paralyzing struggle with anxiety and depression. His symptoms left him socially isolated and though he spoke about desperately wanting to make changes in his life – change jobs, lose weight and go back to school – he felt he could not initiate, never mind sustain any of these pursuits without the presence of a supportive other.

Dennis talked about his relationship with his parents and spoke warmly about how caring they have always been. As he discussed his work in the family lighting business, he gave example after example of times he would become angry and frustrated with both of his parents. As we focused on his difficulty asserting his needs with his parents or expressing his anger, Dennis became acutely aware of how uncomfortable he was in the face of confrontation and conflict. Eventually, we talked about how he sacrificed his authentic responses, in fact, whole parts of himself, in the service of protecting important others from his rage and maintaining an emotional connection with them.

Dennis used the therapeutic relationship with me and Justin to provide the selfobject functions he needed to experience and gradually began to integrate uncomfortable affects such as rage, shame and frustration. He talked to me with Justin by his side, patting him and often remarking that he needed to get a dog as soon as possible. The unconditional love and acceptance that Justin offered was a balm for Dennis as he gingerly began to explore threatening feelings of anger toward the parents he still depended on for much of his emotional sustenance. With Justin's steady supportive presence in the room, Dennis was able to contain his anxiety and give voice to his anger and frustration. As he became more in touch with his rage, Dennis felt seen and valued in the analytic relationship for his ability to experience this thorny affect, rather than for his self-defeating ability to keep his anger under lock and key.

Dennis gradually became significantly less depressed and anxious, enabling him to work consistently and enter into his first intimate relationship with a woman in over twenty years. He began dating via an online site and quickly met Maggie. Unlike his usual easy going, adolescent, somewhat passive social persona, Dennis assumed an adult, almost parental role with his new girlfriend. He supported her financially, counselled her about improving her vocational situation and bemoaned the fact that she was extremely self-involved and unsupportive of his needs.

The paternal, conservative self-state which emerged, an identification with his father, was a new and surprisingly rewarding one for Dennis. While he eschewed most of what smacked of adulthood, i.e. responsibility and commitment, he was beginning to confront his fear of the feelings that both stirred in him. Dennis looked for support and validation as he tentatively stepped into more adult roles. We spoke about the different selves within him, each with his own style and set of priorities and Dennis soaked in the recognition and acceptance that he felt from both Justin and me. With these feelings of approval around his new interpersonal abilities, a more adult Dennis became significantly more engaged in his work and started taking graduate classes in the evening.

As Dennis became able to verbalize his anger and feel empowered and worthy of having a truly intimate, mutual relationship, he ended the relationship with Maggie. This very difficult act reflected his burgeoning ability to embrace conflict and champion his own needs. While he still longs for a significant other, he relies on Justin and me in the treatment to fulfill the mirroring selfobject needs of emotional support, validation and acceptance that his anxious mother, emotionally distant father and impulsive and self-absorbed girlfriend could not provide.

Dennis would come into sessions, saying 'Hey Buddy' as he patted Justin with energy that Justin seemed to enjoy. While he related to me via a maternal transference, he and Justin enjoyed a mutuality that was beneficial to both of them. Dennis was able to give to Justin and to receive from him. This mutuality seemed to be a precursor as well to the shift in his ability to relate from a more adult vantage point and develop more symmetrical and gratifying interpersonal relationships.

Conclusion: a room with a dog

I recently walked into a bakery and grinned knowingly as I read the following sign, 'Chocolate Doesn't Judge, Chocolate Understands'. I believe the dog, like chocolate, induces a visceral sense of understanding, acceptance and belonging. The influence of the quietly powerful dog in relational psychoanalytic treatment is felt in our work's most transformative dimensions: the authenticity and quality of the patient/analyst relationship and the ability of both patient and analyst to access and share the conscious and unconscious intrapsychic experience. As the case examples in this chapter indicate, the dog's accepting and loving presence helps patients feel truly seen and valued, with all of their deficits and demons. Many patients need this feeling of acceptance before they can risk exposing their shame or voicing their split off rage before they are capable of the liberating and empowering experience of authentic emotional relatedness. Similarly, the dog's soothing and holding qualities enhance the analyst's ability to use her own internal experience to navigate the hidden crevices of her patient's internal world. Like a bridge over troubled waters, the dog in the treatment room provides the necessary, if not sufficient ingredients for the unfolding of trust; an unfolding which allows dissociated or buried feelings to reach the restorative shores of the patient/analyst relationship.

References

Benjamin, J. (2012) Intersubjective view of thirdness. *The Psychoanalytic Muse*, Wednesday November 28, 2012.

Boston Change Process Study Group. (2005) The 'Something More' than interpretation revisited: Sloppiness and co-creativity in the analytic encounter. *Journal of American Psychoanalysis*, 53(3), pp. 693–729.

Bromberg, P. (2008) Shrinking the tsunami: Affect regulation, dissociation and the shadow of the flood. *Contemporary Psychoanalysis*, 44(3), pp. 329–350.

Freud, S. (1920). *Introductory lectures on psychoanalysis*. New York and London: W.W. Norton and Company.

Ogden, T. (2004) The analytic third: Implications for psychoanalytic theory and technique. *Psychoanalytic Quarterly*, 73(1), pp. 167–195.

Segal, H. (1964) *Introduction to the work of Melanie Klein*. New York: Basic Books Inc.

Wolf, E. (1988) *Treating the self: Elements of clinical self psychology*. New York and London: The Guilford Press.

13 The secret of grief[1]

Jo Frasca

Harley was Saydee's best friend. He belonged to Saydee's original adoptive family, the Kindly Neighbours across the road. Saydee lived in her sad, emotionally impoverished, violent home and would frequently sit at the gate awaiting the return of her owners and while doing so, watch the comings and goings of her happy, cheerful neighbours. All too often Saydee's owners would not return home; she still dislikes being left alone. Barking incessantly on these occasions she would rouse the Kindly Neighbours from their bed. They would traipse across the road and scoop Saydee up, bringing her into their home where she would snuggle, with Harley, into their warmth and safety. It was Harley she loved most.

Saydee had been living with me for a short time when Harley became unwell and died suddenly. Saydee had been unable to say goodbye to her best friend and as result, for the longest time after Harley's death, Saydee would dash into his home and run to every corner looking for him in all his favourite places. I reflected on her losses, both now and of that of her previous family. If I had a traumatised, lost, little dog before, now after Harley's death, it was far worse. Sadly, Saydee's warm, loving demeanour began to deteriorate before my eyes. Nothing I could do comforted her. She would move away from me when I tried to hold or hug her. She would stare at me from wherever she was, in a disarming manner. At times I felt she thought I had gotten rid of him or wondered why I wasn't bringing him back.

Her shift, noticeable by her posture, her lack of interaction and slower gait, from a buoyant dog to being distracted and lethargic, was palpable. Even her face had a forlorn look as she dragged her head lower. This malaise became so acute that patients began noticing. They began commenting that she appeared to be different. Whereas usually she was out of her basket well before they had even entered the room, tail wagging, now she would remain where she was, in her basket, and look up, as if to acknowledge them, then lie down to sleep. My interpretation was that it was as if she was trying to sleep off the feelings, as we humans are apt to do, a classic symptom of depressive grief.

Around this time, I had been working for about three years, a relatively short time, with a challenging patient, a bright, funny, wiry Irishman. C had explained that he had sought psychotherapy following the transformation he witnessed in his best friend, whom he had met on a rock precipice three decades earlier in Germany. During our initial appointment, he explained that he had recently travelled to Europe to visit his old friend. He told me he had been anxious about the visit because of his friend's constant dark energy. Though he cared deeply about his friend, typically he had found it difficult to spend any length of time with him because, as he frequently said, 'he's so fucking miserable all the time', an experience so anxiety provoking for C that he had contemplated not doing the trip. However, to his shock and pleasure, on this visit, his friend was a delight. His friend opened up in a rare declaration, divulging his own story and his psychotherapy journey. They spoke into the early hours of the morning, his friend sharing some of the darkest things he had learned about himself on his psychotherapy expedition of his life and his family of origin. C described how moving it was to hear how the human body and psyche could mask such detailed important information, then reveal it behaviourally. Though not as overtly dark as his friend, C knew that he too had suffered depression as long as he could recall and had used 'a lot of alcohol and humour' to manage it. They decided that he should embark on a similar journey.

C had waltzed in with the above story and giving me the brief, asked how long 'it' would take. Our three years together were peppered with this theme: 'how long, how long, how long', like a small child on a long car trip, ambivalence reflected in his desire to both stay in psychotherapy and leave. He fluctuated incessantly and almost every session included a reference to 'how long this is taking'.

C appeared never to attach to Saydee. They ignored each other, he not acknowledging her in the room and she not doing her usually patient-specific greeting to acknowledge the entry. This was until one day, when he sailed into the room in his ever-sunny mood and said, 'Eh, what's wrong with yer dog?' I hedged and paused. I looked at him quietly, incredulously, wondering how he knew she was different. C was apt to divert our dialogue in sessions, was tangential, avoidant and dismissive. He was also quite sceptical about 'feelings' and I wondered about the wisdom of explaining Saydee's malaise. On the other hand, I did not want to collude with his avoidant temperament so asked, 'What are you noticing about her?' He did an interesting thing, something I had not witnessed him do before. He looked at her, stared actually, for the longest time, not speaking. I sensed for a time he was no longer aware of his surroundings. Eventually, he looked up from Saydee, apprehension darkening his face. It took on a strange appearance; eyes not blinking, narrowing, his lips white and trembling, his face an ashen shade and his head tilted in a strange position as if stuck in a pose between staring at Saydee and needing to look at me. It was eerie. I had not seen or experienced this level of disquiet from him before. He was usually the epitome of chatty banter and convivial disposition, masking his depression.

Slowly, quietly, with almost-concern, a change from his usual cavalier manner, he said, 'She seems sad, I mean really, really sad'. I felt shocked at his insight. I asked, equally as quietly, so as not to interrupt his process, 'Anything else?' Falteringly he said, 'Like she has lost something, or someone, she loves very much'. We were both quiet again, his gaze going back to Saydee. Unexpectedly, she began to engage with his stare, almost as if they were having a conversation with each other. Suddenly he looked back at me. I was surprised to see tears. I said nothing. I did not want to disrupt his connection with Saydee. She was clearly evoking some long-lost memory for him. I felt any word uttered from my lips right now, at this moment, would interfere with his internal process and recall and might catapult him back to his defence mechanism and avoidance, and I would have the chatty, bolshy Irishman back in the room.

It appeared he could no longer tolerate what he was experiencing. Neither could he look at me. He was staring down at a place somewhere between his feet, arms resting on his thighs. Saydee settled back into her basket, perhaps assessing the loss of his attention, and not appearing to particularly care. I waited, saying nothing. It was quiet. I then noted a wet stain on his knee, dark against the fabric of his jeans. Tear drops. His hunched shoulders begin to tremble. Finally, a sound escaped from his quivering lips. He answered my question, 'Death'. He was then wracked with sobs, for the longest time, all the while hiding his face in his hands. Tears, snot and drool escaped through his fingers. Suddenly he screamed, 'Why did she have to die? Why? Why? Why? I didn't mean it'. I was momentarily startled, though not as much as Saydee. I can usually intervene with a hand movement to stop her from approaching a patient. The hand movement did not work on that day. She sprung from her bed into his lap in what appeared to be one single bound. Briefly, I had an opportunity to experience remorse, for allowing her to get so close to him during what appeared to be a catharsis of archaic, painful and probably traumatic memories. But he grabbed her, almost roughly, and held her close, sobbing into her fur. Now they were both covered in tears, snot and drool, neither appearing to care. He was repeating, 'Yes, yes, yes, you know, you know, I know you know'. Rocking back and forth, Saydee allowing him to hold her in a way she would never have tolerated from me. I waited.

Eventually, his torrent subsided, his grip on Saydee loosened. She nestled close to him, appearing to know she needed to be near, both seeming to want to be near each other. This was familiar territory for her, though not for him. He told of the tragic loss of his mother when he was young. He told a story of the death of a girlfriend at age sixteen. He said he had told no one, shared nothing about how responsible he felt for both deaths. His mother crashed the car; he was the four-year-old passenger. His girlfriend drowned after he had begged her not to go into the raging, swirling eddy. He asked about Saydee. I told him the abridged version of Harley's recent death. He picked her up again from the couch near him, holding her close, saying, 'Aye, it hurts doesn't it, girl?'

Finally, he stops complaining about how long it is taking. Finally, he understands why it takes so long. He also begins to understand why the drugs, incarceration, rehabilitation units, electroconvulsive therapy (ECT) and cognitive behaviour therapy as treatments, and his use of alcohol, have not worked to cure him of 'this depression'. It had been grief all along. Allowing him now to delve into his history enabled him to become attached to the work, to the psychotherapist and to the dog, his fear of our deaths and his losses all floridly filling the room. He and Saydee become pals. I don't call her off when he goes into catharsis. He has contracted with me to let her up near him at those times. He says it is a comfort to have her tap at him and for some reason, it helps him get more deeply in touch with his grief. Finally, our work has begun.

As the patient's own grief was not forthcoming in the early stages of our work pre-Saydee's intervention, I was left to hypothesis why he had not processed that grief around the death of his mother. He knew his father had been so grief-stricken as to not work for years; his father's grief took precedence over the four-year old's grieving process. In confirmation of this, he recalled conversations with a paternal aunt saying, 'yes your father nearly died of grief after your mother was killed; we knew you were too young to fully understand so we were all focused on his recovery'. The telling of this part of his story evoked the patient's rage at the neglect of his right to grieve his dead mother and spoke to Peskin's (2019) thinking that '... the highly ranked mourners may appropriate another's grief by claiming a stronger sense of entitlement' and that 'the self is injured when one's right to grieve is withheld, overlooked or otherwise curtailed by others' (p. 477). My hope was that in Saydee liberating his grief he might find that, 'grief is most[ly] our own when we protest it's being taken from us' (ibid). I hoped this might be his first step toward recovery in our now overt work on his mother's death where he began protesting and raging about not being allowed to grieve in preference to his father.

Freud (1917, ibid) in Mourning and Melancholia, contends that in deferring grief, one is in fact 'resisting to give up the lost object' perhaps explaining the two levels in which this patient resisted his grief: one where he was not assisted in expressing his grief and the second, where it was in fact deferred to the others' 'more important' grieving process.

In ascertaining Saydee's part in his release of long-standing grief, I refer to Peskin's insight about how difficult, if not impossible, it is for people to process grief without the witnessing or recognition of other or community. He explains further that grief can be stymied when there is a threat, as was the case with this patient's expressed fear that his father might also die, a fear that would keep him quiet and compliant. In those protracted periods where the person does not grieve, we might understand that this patient was ridiculed or refused the right to grieve, an embargo which can precipitate emotional sustainability, hence creating a protective shell that fends off any opportunity for exposure of feelings (Bowlby, 1980). The more the child is denied their grief, the more anxiety and distress escalate and become habitual (ibid). The extent to which C deflects is tangential, adds humour and drinks excessively is perhaps an indication of how he managed significant levels of anxiety and distress. If the negation of feelings continues on the part of both the family and the child, the child is then unlikely to see the grief as significant or even to acknowledge its existence (ibid). It was when his grief was at this level that this patient found his way into psychotherapy.

Bowlby's (ibid) formula for healthy development in a child who experiences the early death of a parent includes the following ingredients: the hope that, prior to the death of the parent, the child had a securely attached relationship; that following the death, the surviving parent and extended family give timely and truthful information to the child; that the child is permitted questions, not only about that parent's death but about death generally; the child is included in the surviving parent's own grief process; and that the surviving parent creates an environment of security, reassurance and solace for the grieving child. As if to illustrate Bowlby's formula, C would repeatedly lament, 'Why didn't they talk to me about her death, or let me talk about it?' He believed that, had he been able to talk and ask questions about what happened to his mother, he may not have felt responsible and guilty for her death.

C had always felt responsible for his mother's death, simply by virtue of the fact that he happened to be in the car at the time. It was years before he could hear his own words, 'Her death had nothing to do with me'.

Bromberg (2011) tells us that is it somewhat normal for the brain, in dealing with 'disjunctive truths' (pp. 98–101), to activate dissociation. He also contends that the fear of emotional dysregulation can cause this level of dissociation (Bromberg, 2008). When the situation is extremely traumatic, such as the death of a parent, the brain will protect us from the 'emotionally threatening situation' (ibid). It is when this 'unbearable' level of dissociation is present that there can be developmental damage affecting human to human connection.

I was left with many questions about how this patient was able to use Saydee as a portal to his traumatic grief. Was there a void in the very transference and countertransference that was required to liberate the trauma (Maroda, 1998)? Was it rather Saydee's loss of Harley that triggered C's repressed grief, a process I was unable to engage within my griefless self-state? Did Saydee's empathic eye-locking gaze allow him the experience of finally being seen and felt in a way that undermined his defences against his long-held grief? Did Saydee take over the position of the psychotherapist in appearing responsive and attuned?

Bromberg (in Mitchell and Aron, 1999) contends that it is incumbent on the psychotherapist not only to allow, and even encourage, the enactment to occur, but also to participate in it. I believe that C and I were engaged in an enactment, whereby I was perhaps experienced by C as not unlike his father and aunt, who, by failing to countenance his grief, ensured its continued disavowal. Saydee, conversely, rather than complicit with the patient in this disavowal, somehow created a relational milieu conducive to a shared or twinship experience. Not only did Saydee's gifts to C of her responsive, empathic attunement and an experience of shared subjectivities grant him an alternative to his more familiar experience – that of his subjectivity having been colonised by his father (and possibly, by extension, me) – but also as the third in the room, Saydee interrupted the enactment in which C and I were inadvertently engaged. These two offerings by Saydee provided to C the opportunity to repeal, or even liberate, his defences and generate a process of developmental repair.

Despite the temptation, when I find myself in unknown territory, to bolster my doubt with interpretations or interventions informed by theories of the unconscious (Bromberg, ibid), I allowed our work to transition into an alternative mode, and onto the foreign landscape upon which we, in the room, all found ourselves thereby, ironically, allowing the therapeutic work to unfold between Saydee and C.

With Bowlby's steps for healthy development following the death of a parent in mind, I would like to think that Saydee had at some level given him the empathy and permission that no-one else (including this psychotherapist) had and thereby finally allowed him to express grief.

In conclusion, I suggest that depression, trauma, dissociation, enactment and grief are not always organised in such a manner to which the psychotherapist can apply a prescription for the integration. Saydee's interaction with the patient demonstrated unmistakeably that when grief meets grief or the patient feels seen in a necessary manner, or if the psychotherapist is attuned, it can often be the most unexpected event or environment in the room that will liberate the patient's story.

Note

1 This chapter has been adapted from *Delving Deeper: Understanding Diverse Approaches While Exploring Psychotherapy* by Jo Frasca, self-published in 2016.

References

Bowlby, J. (1980) *Attachment and loss volume 3: Loss sadness and depression*. London: Hogarth Press and the Institute of Psychoanalysis.

Bromberg, P. (2008) Shrinking the tsunami: Affect regulation, dissociation and the shadow of the flood. *Contemporary Psychoanalysis*, 44(3), pp. 329–350.

Bromberg, P. (2011) *The shadow of the tsunami: And the growth of the relational mind*. New York and Oxon: Routledge.

Maroda, K. (1998) *Seduction, surrender, and transformation: Emotional engagement in the analytic process*. Mahwah, NJ: The Analytic Press.

Mitchell, S.A., and Aron, L. (1999) *Relational psychoanalysis: The emergence of a tradition*. New York and London: Routledge.

Peskin, H. (2019) Who has the right to mourn?: Relational deference and the ranking of grief. *Psychoanalytic Dialogues*, 29(4), pp. 477–492.

14 The conduit to fear and anger, and the story[1]

Jo Frasca

Story 1

Z could barely speak. Not because she was mute but because she was un-questionably traumatised and suffering PTSD from domestic violence and had been diagnosed with chronic depression, a feeling she described as 'grinding life to a halt'. Much of what we did in session was around parenting issues. She had had a baby at a young age and, predictably, her own lack of being appropriately parented had created a deficit in her ability to parent her own child. She frequently struggled to know the correct course of action in raising her baby. Greenberg and Mitchell (1983), and Mitchell and Aron (1999) described that when early development is contaminated by traumatic life (in this case domestic violence) the child learns to dissociate so that they can, at least at some level, remain attached to the parental figure and preserve their internal world. As the violence continues it exacerbates the dissociative mechanisms which are then strengthened by splitting off parts of the self. In this case not speaking was a part of her split-off self. She not only needed to stay attached but she needed to find a safe way to do so, and by being mute, quiet and cowering from the violence, it assisted her attachment, lest any vestiges of parenting evaporate. In this way, the child develops a self that relates increasingly to the dissociative part of their world than to the real world, shaping a way of being and the attachment that continues to plague relationships throughout their lives (ibid). It appeared, however, that Doogie would not be a trigger to this dissociative part.

Our contract was clear. She wanted to work on the feelings of depression that pervaded her life, though doing this seems almost impossible with her. She could barely find words and frequently felt that, because she did not talk, her time in psychotherapy was useless and she berated herself for 'not doing psychotherapy properly'. Our focus became about her daughter and in that, we were able to stay connected and build enough trust to deepen the work – perhaps a steppingstone to us locating the source of depression. While comforted in the knowledge that even in that more cognitive framework, we would have been doing significant work.

It is frequently difficult for traumatised people to tell any part of their story. Not because they are intentionally withholding but because it is deeply hidden, especially from them. Staying in and working with the resistance with patients can be, on the one hand, difficult work, and on the other, rewarding. It is often a time where we are able to build the psychotherapist-patient relationship and the waiting may allow the unconscious to unfurl. In an attempt to normalise the process I might say, 'it could be that we possibly sit together, indefinitely, if you can bear it.' or I might take the time to explain that during this time we could be doing important things like developing awareness and building trust.

One important consideration underpinning my treatment plan at all times with patients and is a helpful reminder when the work is slow and appears not to be advancing is that our material is usually deeply buried, embedded and entrenched arcanely in the unconscious history that it is has become a part of the fabric of our everyday life; we barely know of its existence, and thus not easily found.

On one particular day, Z uncharacteristically waltzed into the room with zeal, even opening the conversation. 'You have a dog?' This time, I managed to avoid a frame-panic as discussed in Chapter 10, and decided to introduce her to my then canine, Doogie; it was then that our work was to take a dramatic turn. In that first session after I allowed Doogie into the room, the patient slid off the couch onto the floor beside him and patting him, began a dialogue. Her session content transformed from that day forward. Each session began with a 'hello' greeting to Doogie, and an enquiry about how he was and what he had been up to. She sometimes shared with him an account of her week or an interaction which I coveted. Doogie was eliciting more than I had ever been able to find or extract from those lips. Perhaps she was creating a *carom-style* communication (Woollams and Brown, 1979; see Chapter 10, this volume). As Doogie sat with her I began to hear stories to which I had not been privy prior to his arrival in the room. She had had a lovely time with her daughter at the park (which unexpectedly included details of the various pieces of equipment on which they played); she had been angry with her mother for bullying her; she was frightened of her successful sister; her father had visited. Rarely, if ever, did I receive news of father. I did not overtly use this information for quite some time. I felt that dialogue was between her and Doogie and I was careful not to thwart that process. With such rich dialogue filling the therapeutic space, I found myself excited. Finally, I was given permission to work with aspects of this information. I knew it was still a dialogue between her and Doogie and that I had, at some level been tentatively invited in, though it appeared in a sort-of interloper role. In an attempt to not invade her world with Doogie, initially, I would frame most questions with something like, 'I heard you tell Doogie the other day ...' We did a lot of work in this way. Eventually, I was allowed to receive the information by way of more direct, first-hand, dialogue. The patient would stroke Doogie continually and speak back, though still conferring with him occasionally. Doogie had become the conduit for a powerful, painful history to emerge, her damaged past weaving its way into the room; violent beatings to her mother, herself and her sister by the husband and father, so bad, on occasion, she feared death, which now she shared openly with me.

A dark account of her life leaped into the room with wild, vivid imagery. It was in the talking that she 'heard' her own words, through that narrative with Doogie. As the words wove their way into the room, she was able to see the travesty happening at home. Sessions became difficult, mostly due to her never having been able to recall aspects of the story which were now pouring out. The awareness and release of such a traumatic history, in her own words, her own narrative, distressed her. She was tormented as she spoke, but keep the story flowing from session to session. We were simultaneously processing the story and her relationship to the story – and how frightening that was to her. Despite her trepidation, she admitted to frequently experiencing relief after sessions. Eventually, she shared that she had had no idea her story would come out in this manner. I will admit to being in awe of what was happening. I had never worked in this unorthodox manner and was struck by the power of it. Our work had changed. Doogie had liberated her story and a painful history found a way to materialise and to be heard and acknowledged, by both of us. Furthermore, she reported behavioural change in her day to day life. She came into sessions with an awareness of how she had managed what would normally have been a rage-filled situation with her daughter, mother, sister, father, anyone. She knew something was finally shifting.

It feels important to declare that at the time I did not have the confidence as an early practicing psychotherapist to have conversations and theoretical dialogue with colleagues about working in such an untraditional manner. I knew it was irregular. It was the late 90s and I could find very little written on the subject. Instead, I fell back on the primary premise, the cornerstone of the helping professions, 'do no harm' and although I did not know anyone else working in this way, I felt it appropriate for this patient. I thus rigorously, perhaps even obsessively, documented every moment of every session, knowing I would need a record if this unconventional way of working was questioned at any point. Years later, when I did finally begin sharing aspects of working in this way, I had varying responses. By then I did not have the same level of fear from the potential critics, and this patient was thriving.

Eventually, we finished our work together. She felt 'done'. The depression no longer had a hold on her life. She was managing well. I did not hear from her for a long time. Around seven years post-treatment termination I received a simple text message, 'I often think of Doogie, you and our work. My daughter and I are happy and have moved to the ocean away from Mum and my sister. How is Doogie?' To which I replied, 'It's good to hear from you. I am touched you have made contact, and that you are both happy. I know you will be sad to read this, but Doogie died. I guess his work here was done'. Some days later she replied, 'I cried, but I guessed he might have died. I know you are okay because you know how to deal with things. I do better now thanks to all of our work back then'.

I guess when I brought Saydee into the room I was holding onto this unique experience.

Story 2

A long-term patient, R came to session, previously having been ambivalent about Doogie's presence in the room. On this particular occasion Doogie got up to greet him, then sauntered back to his favourite position on the floor. The patient appeared significantly agitated. He laughed his familiar hyena-style laugh, a laugh he used to avoid the pain of what was circulating around his psyche. Today's laugh felt more fearful, severe. With unusual precise clarity, he said, 'It might be a good idea if you don't have the dog in the room today because I'm not sure what I might do'. R was predisposed to rage-filled outbursts, though not often in the room. Mostly they arrive through the telling of his story. At those times I would attempt to process what he thought or feared might happen around the outbursts. On this day, I complied and removed Doogie. I knew this was not a turf fight for my attention, nor was it a superfluous request, the patient was ashen and trembling. Something was going on and it felt imperative to assist in alleviating any external stressors. Playing a reflective psychotherapist right now did not feel like a good intervention. I returned to the room, sat down and waited. I waited a few moments, so the patient knew my interaction with Doogie was over. I maintained eye contact with him so that he would know I was fully present, present in the way we both knew he needed. Eventually, I said, softly, 'Bad isn't it?' His face crumpled at that moment and he began crying. He cried for most of that session. I let him cry for as long as the session allowed as this was indeed a rare event. I was also relieved, in hindsight, that I had not attempted to process why he wanted Doogie out of the room. Had I done so, it would have cut across his immediate need and the issue at hand. I realised that in him asking me to remove the object and exiling the dog, he appeared freer to demonstrate his distress. Historically expressing distress, articulating fear and having a request were all challenges for him, so I wondered whether the act of responding immediately to his request might have aided his connectivity to this emotion. Hoffman in Mitchell and Aron (1999) suggests that if the psychotherapist is able to communicate (verbally and or behaviourally) in the sense that they are acting in an approachable, kindly manner, useful transference can occur, and the patient is more likely to respond positively. And while this work is not about positive reinforcement or arousing positive states, on this occasion the patient was in need of an experience of the psychotherapist taking his needs seriously. Bromberg (2011) extends this thinking in that the psychotherapist's own need to have clarity of a certain situation (i.e. why he needed the dog out of the room) can in fact create resistance in the patient.

Towards the end of this session, being careful not to abruptly severe his process, I said that we didn't have much time left and that it might useful for us to debrief a little.

Hunched over, a position he had occupied for most of this session, he cried a little longer, which I was relieved about; rather than complying, which was more typical, today he was just in the feeling, doing what he needed.

Eventually, he looked at me and leaned back on the couch, as if needing support to be upright. Speaking softly he explained that for the first time in our work together he was able to reflect on his 'damaged' childhood, his 'horrid' flashbacks, his grief at having been 'neglected' and that his awareness that these unbearable features were the triggers to his 'out of control' behaviours.

He said, 'I didn't know how I was going to tell you all that has happened, and now I'm out of time. And I didn't know if I was going to be angry, because I usually am …'. He trailed off and stopped. After a long pause, we arranged another session that week, agreeing that he needed more time and support. Hesitating he asked if he had time to see Doogie before leaving. This was most unusual; he rarely had a request. I had a brief moment to consider the likelihood of a significant intrapsychic change in him making such an appeal. This was his second verbal request today. I went to the door to call Doogie knowing he would not be too far away. Sauntering into the room he went straight over to the patient, standing at his feet.

The patient looked up at me and said, 'He's telling me he knows it was okay that I kicked him out of the room today'. I didn't know what Doogie was saying, but whatever the patient interpreted at that moment was fine by me. He had brought some important archaic memories and trauma and I was grateful for the canine help. He said, 'Thank you Doogie, you helped me say how bad it was today and your Mum got it immediately!' While we chuckled together, 'Doogie's Mum' also got that this patient's range of emotions was so limited and confused he barely knew the difference between fear, grief, sadness, anger and anything in between. For now, he had experienced all of these, disguised as anger, and had taken another step forward.

Clinical reflections

I wonder what the outcome might have been for both patients without the assistance of the canine. In both cases, it seemed that the canine liberated some aspects of their archaic repressed histories. Did the canine precipitate the shift? Was it the third that elicited the patients' projections? And helped them to articulate previously unspoken words?

Both patients had experienced significant trauma and had developed a minimally affective ability to connect relationally, with family, friends and the psychotherapist. The ongoing and often insurmountable struggle in the room was their ability to dissociate, a dissociation that had erased their knowledge of the enormity of their own trauma. It is easy to discount the effect of trauma by identifying it as anxiety. Bromberg (2011) discusses the significant differing machination of anxiety versus trauma by describing that 'traumatic affect is not anxiety with its volume turned up' (p. 49). He identifies that in the case of trauma the brain is left with 'unprocessed, dissociated affect'. It is within this sphere that each patient was in a relationship with their world.

What does become difficult in this traumatic state is how to engage with the dissociated parts that arrive in the room. Trauma is expressed in various ways and enters our practices overtly through behaviour and language. That story which is not spoken or symbolised is an enigma, leaving the need for greater interpretive work. Or does it? We may be tempted to recruit our knowledge and theory and attempt to make an interpretation or produce a story from the information that we have been privy to. McGleughlin (2015, p. 215) urges the psychotherapist to 'unlearn' how we interpret and understand trauma which manifests without language. She says in our need to know, name and give meaning to the patient's trauma we may misinterpret, misrepresent or worse, violate that person's experience. In her (2015) paper McGleughlin gives a small but beautiful rendition of dialogue between the patient and herself. She describes herself as 'cringing' as she shares a dialogue, where she illuminates a conversation between herself and a patient, a conversation marked by her attempts to interpret the words of a traumatised patient and the consequences of this intervention (p. 219). She explains that the ensuing conversation is less about resistance and more about the patient's fear that the psychotherapist might see some unbearable truth in that interpretation. I believe that whatever I might have said, in this first example here, was un-hearable for her, while somehow, Doogie did not pose that same threat. And in that lack of threat (and knowledge that Doogie would not be doing interpretations) the traumatic story, together with her dissociated parts, were able to weave their way into the room.

McGleughlin (ibid, p. 215) uses the term 'negative enactment', where we have permission to feel the absence of doing, or knowing, what the trauma is about and the work becoming more about holding any insightful interpretations in a conscious place but doing nothing with it, a sort of unlearning what we know about trauma and its effects. In doing so she believes we are better able to learn (as opposed to 'know') what is happening in these traumatic spaces for our patients, thus allowing more space for the trauma to arrive in its own way and at its own pace. She suggests that the knowing and using of words is not yet possible.

McGleughlin (2015) explains her process of not being interpretive, or unlearning, using negative enactment by her use of, 'a collage of different experiences, atmospheres, registers, and voices … to convey my process of psychoanalytic witness to trauma' (p. 215). I was left to wonder whether, where McGleughlin used images in the form of photographs to engage and stimulate her patient, I was similarly a witness to trauma – revealed by the entry into or indeed exit from the room of a canine, a third. While the photographs utilised in her work were used as a platform to understand the trauma, they did trigger and haunt both the patient and the psychotherapist. I wondered if both Doogie's presence with one patient, and his removal with the other, in some way triggered memories and behaviour for each of them, allowing their own haunting pasts into consciousness. There was a point in which I felt, in both cases, having the animal as the third gave permission for that 'negative enactment'. Furthermore, in not needing to process those moments, canine in, canine out, and by acting from the less threatening, unlearned position in that non-interpretive way, the trauma was allowed to be suspended between us all.

In the second case described above, it appeared Doogie's presence in the room elicited both the patient's fear of his behaviour towards the dog and an imperative to protect him. In removing Doogie and with him, the fear that had previously rendered R inactive, R was unshackled from his protective impulse, thereby decontaminating the space and enabling him to locate, then express, feelings to which he had previously had no access.

And did the communication to remove the dog from the room, further prevent and downgrade the patient's own anticipated rage outburst making way for grief? Bromberg (2011) suggests that if traumatised patients can experience, from the psychotherapist, the psychotherapist's subjective experience, the patient may eventually be able to relate to the intersubjectivity between them. In such moments the patient may possibly have the experience of identifying their own dysfunctions and limitations and be less likely triggered into a dissociative state (ibid). In the same way, it may be possible that a traumatised patient's experience of a dog's unconditional love is in fact borne out of an understanding which their intersubjectivity is unveiled. Bromberg (ibid) uses the concept of 'mentalisation' to explain that when two people are not able to connect intersubjectively a sort of deadlock occurs. In introducing Doogie did I release the deadlock and in effect liven the intersubjectivity that I was unable to previously evoke, thereby reviving the patient's relatedness in the room? Was it the interaction with the dog that allowed some aspect of liberation of feelings? In Bromberg's narrative, the patient was finally able to experience themselves through the eyes (or relatedness) of another.

Interestingly, the dog appeared to have created a sense of safety, for Z by his presence, and for R, by having been removed. Regardless, both seemed to relate to Doogie as a less threatening entity, his presence – or indeed absence – being therapeutically useful and perhaps a significant, contributing factor in allowing improvement in the relationship with the psychotherapist

Bromberg draws from the amusing and clever movie *Analyse This*, to offer a rich explanation of how the dynamic of 'negotiating between collisions' (ibid, p. 53) can shift the relatedness in the room and becomes the key factor in therapeutic change. 'Negotiating between collisions' refers to the phenomenon whereby the psychotherapist enters into the 'collision between subjectivities' (ibid) and means that we need to stay in touch with what is changing, shifting and moving with the patient, moment to moment and session to session. I felt there might have been something lacking in my own capacity to 'negotiate collisions'. Perhaps I was too empathic, too conciliatory, even too interpretive. Did I lack the capacity to permit intersubjectivity thereby creating a sort of lifelessness in a relationship that required relationality? And did my own dissociative process influence both patients so that they were still able to not only dissociate to a large degree in session but that they were able to discount that level of dissociation?

In conclusion, I defer again to McGleughlin (2015) who cautions that in attempting to name or make too much literal sense of the trauma, we can in fact create an experience unfaithful to the patient's inner traumatic world. With the use of a canine, this stumbling block appears somewhat to have been bypassed. Perhaps an animal creates a conduit to humans to access and express previously inaccessible information, creating enough of a human-nonhuman relationship for change to occur.

Note

1 This chapter has been adapted from *Delving Deeper: Understanding Diverse Approaches While Exploring Psychotherapy* by Jo Frasca, self-published in 2016.

References

Bromberg, P. (2011) *The shadow of the tsunami: And the growth of the relational mind.* New York and Oxon: Routledge.

Greenberg, J.R., and Mitchell, S.A. (1983) *Object relations in psychoanalytic theory.* Cambridge, MA: Harvard University Press.

McGleughlin, J. (2015) Do we find or loose ourselves in the negative? *Psychoanalytic Dialogue.* vol. 25, no. 2, pp. 214–236.

Mitchell, S.A., and Aron, L. (1999) Relational psychoanalysis: The emergence of a tradition. New York and London: Routledge.

Woollams, S., and Brown, M. (1979) *The total handbook of transactional analysis.* Upper Saddle River, NJ: Prentice Hall.

15 Together, we can find your voice. Love, Phoebe

Lynn Higgins

The treatment

With long blond unkempt hair that was cascading around and covering her face, Abby entered while steadfastly looking down and towards the floor. She was clutching onto her book for dear life as she shuffled ever so slowly into my office. She sat in the middle of the large couch looking as if she folded into the middle of it, not daring to look up from her lap. Sitting there, she looked as though the couch was both swallowing and consuming her. Phoebe immediately jumped up, without any hesitation and curled up next to her. Abby, saying nothing, was glued to the pages in front of her which she turned slowly, trying to manage whatever she was feeling and whatever might be going through her mind. A small, ten-pound Boston Terrier with big brown eyes and a loving and sensitive disposition, Phoebe remained curled up next to Abby on that couch. Phoebe was just not moving. As I tried to offer some conversation with her, where she was, and what we do here, Phoebe sighed and placed her head on Abby's lap. As Abby was looking up at me, she placed her hand on Phoebe's head and left it there.

Little did I know that this would be the beginning of something significant and special that would occur between the two of them and the three of us. For the next few months as we became accustomed to each other, this pattern of Phoebe gently but obviously placing her head on Abby's lap as they settled in on the couch, would occur towards the beginning of each session. As time went on this beginning became a kind of ritual where Abby would wait for Phoebe to jump up next to her. At some point, the content of the sessions became secondary to what was developing on the couch.

As a seven-year-old girl Abby was not social—as opposed to anti-social. She wanted desperately to be included in groups during lunch, play, anything with the other kids at school. She would laugh awkwardly and say things the other kids clearly didn't understand. She was so painfully inappropriate that she was consistently ignored or rejected and called weird by almost everyone she came in contact with. She was excluded from most activities and not chosen for groups or teams causing her to retreat further into her own world. She was lost for hours in this private place and became less meaningfully verbal.

She wasn't eating or sleeping, so she would go to school tired and hungry, but unaware of her hunger. The fact that Abby was not eating, yet hungry for contact from others, left me almost aching for how starving she must have truly been. She was very thin and looked rather gangly and waif-like. Her attachment to others and her interest in life felt aloof, distant and cut off. She wanted everything to do with people, and nothing, protecting herself from persistent rejection by her own distancing. It was at this point, at the school's recommendation, that her mother brought her in for treatment.

Abby has a twin brother who has severe autism. To this day, he is not toilet trained and is nonverbal. He spends much of his time with his maternal grandparents because their mother cannot manage both of them. For the first four years of Abby's life, her mother suffered from severe post-partum depression and could not care for either Abby or her brother—at all. As a result, both Abby and her brother lived with their maternal grandparents exclusively for those first four years. Her father, drug-addicted, and also not involved, passed away when she was three years old. As her mother clawed her way out of her depression, she began medication, therapy and entered social work school to help her understand herself and her children. She wanted to become a better mother, a present mother. She subsequently met a man, David, who loves all of them dearly. He presents as rather naïve with little insight and complains that he doesn't earn respect in his endeavors, but he has a heart of gold and the best of intentions when it comes to both Abby's mother and her children.

Mom, David and Abby would come to the weekly sessions and sit in the waiting room. Phoebe would greet them all, especially Abby. Abby would wait for Phoebe to trot into the treatment room ahead of her, follow her and they would resume their positions on the couch. Abby would draw, read her books, play with her Gameboy. She would, it seemed out of obligation, introduce me to what she was playing but remained so focused and engrossed in her play that my presence seemed inconsequential.

With Phoebe sitting between us on the couch, out of desperation one day, I began to 'use' Phoebe to communicate with Abby. I said, 'I did NOT hear Abby say that Phoebe!!' And then—for Phoebe—in a rather loud and astonishing voice, 'WHAT?' I would continue in this manner until one day Abby looked up and responded with, 'What did Phoebe just say I said?' So, I playfully responded with, '"Phoebe said you really want Lynn to sit right next to you"'. Or, 'Phoebe said, "You really want Lynn to play with you."' Abby would vehemently disagree with Phoebe that she said anything of the kind, but at least she was responding and talking. She began correcting Phoebe. I felt like I had struck gold. I would slightly exaggerate my responses until she would laugh and correct me to make sure I said whatever it was that she meant, exactly as she meant it. This initial commentary back and forth was playful, light, silly and a bit provocative. She then began to ask Phoebe to tell me something that felt to me like a feeling or something she was trying to communicate. We were beginning to use Phoebe as the medium to both communicate and to clarify what she was feeling. All the while, Phoebe would sit next to Abby with her head on her lap, seemingly unaware of what was playing out around her, but steadfast in her presence.

As this dynamic unfolded and developed, the atmosphere in the room became much more playful and spontaneous. Abby began to bring in a giant stuffed bear named Bear-y that she had had at home, which soon was accompanied by a plethora of additional stuffed animals. Each week she would lug multiple stuffed animals into the room, introduce them to me, set them up along the furniture and make them talk in the same way that I was talking to her through Phoebe. They spoke to each other, to Phoebe, to me, and back to her, about children at school, about her mother, about anything. Over time, not only did these conversations develop in their content, but they also became more thoughtful, contemplative, reflective and fluent. Phoebe always had a say about a situation. 'She' asked questions about families, games on the playground, and how children talk to each other. Abby insisted these conversations continue at home so we both taught her mom how to be part of the dynamic with her stuffed bears. Her mom was thus able to develop a real communication with Abby. As this continued over a period of about a year, Abby's voice began to change as she would jump out of the role of talking like one of the bears or Phoebe and would use her own voice to correct them. She began to use her voice in such a way that I was then able to ask her questions and remark more directly.

Abby began to write story after story, both in session and out of session. She had so much to say. Her stories were about children on the playground, children not listening to each other and groups of children playing together happily, about music class that felt extremely uncomfortable, about having a sibling that was disliked and who was the character in her story of whom she felt painfully ashamed. These stories launched many conversations about social dynamics as well as her internal wishes and feelings. Conversations would happen either directly or through Phoebe, but importantly, they began to happen.

At home, Abby was becoming belligerent and angry. She wasn't listening to her mother and they were fighting constantly. She refused to shower, eat, and do her homework. She was at risk of failing math, in particular. Index cards were used, games were played, but Abby refused to engage with anything to do with math. During this period, her mom would come in periodically for some sessions alone to discuss ways in which she could encourage Abby to express her anger verbally and modify how she was responding to Abby. This period was extremely challenging for both Abby and her mom, in different ways. Abby became so angry that she felt inaccessible both in session to me and to some extent at home to her mom. However, this was less the case with Phoebe; at some point, Phoebe sat so close to Abby that Abby had no choice but to respond to her. This went on for many weeks until Abby began talking to and through Phoebe again, in ways that were reminiscent of an earlier period. We went back to square one.

Again, slowly she became more responsive to me. 'Phoebe' began asking her about her feelings of rejection by kids at school. She had a lot to say about what was happening socially at this point. She told Phoebe about feeling weird, about not being like other kids and feeling like she had no friends, even though everybody else did. She told Phoebe everything that was happening in school. 'Phoebe' listened and I, like Phoebe, commented in ways that let Abby know she was seen and heard by her.

Abby also had a teacher who really cared about her, who helped her navigate everything from negotiating conflicts with other children to how to join games on the playground during recess. She had Abby come in for extra help with math and spoke to her mother about getting her some new clothes that were more appropriate and that would help her fit in—at least in terms of looking more like her peers. Abby began to care about her appearance and also to notice what she did to put other children off that had earned her the label, weird. She began to modify her behavior. She began to care about math as well as her other subjects. She also wanted to have clothes more like those the other children were wearing. This made a huge difference in other children's reactions to her.

Abby began to like to sing in the chorus class. Her teacher encouraged her to try out for the school play, a musical. She got a part with a one-line solo and as a moderate lead. She worked hard to learn her lines and to develop her stage presence. She had to learn to use her voice loud enough so that she was able to project out toward the audience—so she could be heard. Although awkward, she began to fit in with the other children. Having to project her voice in this way helped her find the strength that had been already percolating within her. She excelled. Her grades improved. She began reaching out socially and writing her own stories, complex stories about real issues. She won an award for her stories, which helped her gain visibility and acknowledgment for something important to her. At the end of sixth grade, Abby was solidly on her way to experiencing herself differently in this world.

Theoretical considerations

When Abby walked into the treatment room as a young seven-year-old, it was clear she was severely depressed, cut off and hesitant. It seemed that she hardly existed. I felt as if I was sitting alone in the room—clearly an empathic experience of what Abby had been feeling. Altman et al. (2010) discuss the importance of the relational therapist's countertransferential experiences as a mechanism for honing-in on the goings-on in the family through empathy towards both the child and the parent/family. Paying attention to the parent-child interaction, listening to descriptions of experiences at home and one's own affective responses—all inform the direction a therapist will move.

Stern discusses the infant's repeated and yet unsuccessful 'attempts to invite and solicit the mother that fail to bring her to life [and] ... to be with her by way of identification and imitation' (1995, p. 100). Abby had learned to survive by 'suppressing her own perceptions and feelings [taking into herself] ... the parental badness in order to hold onto the security of believing [s]he has a good parent' (Altman et al., 2010, p. 84). Modell (in Kohon, 1999) refers to Andre Green's concept of the *dead mother syndrome* as a fundamental and as a 'traumatic disruption in maternal relatedness in infancy and early childhood' (p. 76), which potentially serves as the seat of early trauma. The subsequent deadening becomes 'clothing' we wear and carry with us each day and throughout life. Abby desperately needed contact with her mother, so she 'deadened' herself in order to survive and to maintain an illusion of contact with her mother, connecting with the emotionally absent mother in order to find some way to feel some aliveness through the contact, even if it meant maintaining a chronic deadness. This 'imitation may be the only way the infant can engage the mother. If I cannot be loved by mother, I will become her' (Kohon, 1999, p. 78). Abby had 'taken in' and become an earlier, depressed version of her mother.

Stern describes a depressed mother as physically present and emotionally absent because 'she can no longer or hasn't been able to engage or remain engaged with or become emotionally invested in her child' (1995, p. 99). It seemed that all Abby's mother's long-held fantasies about repairing, connecting or redoing her own childhood that she may once have felt, were stuck and thus transmitted to Abby. Stern suggests that when the mother relinquishes such fantasies they become replaced by the reality of the disappointments in her childhood. 'The accompanying profound sense of loss that runs beneath the sense of worlds gained' (Stern, 1995, p. 25). Therefore, the profound sense of loss and sadness that Abby's mother has carried with her, which was then enacted and communicated to Abby, may have then contributed to her profound and lasting post-partum depression.

Altman et al. discuss the need for the parent to recognize the child's inner world, without which s/he feels 'alone and [with] a part of himself that he cannot make sense of. Recognition, then, allows the child to feel real and part of the world' (2010, p. 85). Abby had not only become the badness she felt from her mother but had also been disappearing from any sense of aliveness.

Abby was thus extremely cautious and clear about not wanting to relate to me or anyone else for that matter. However, she tolerated Phoebe by allowing her to sidle up and sit next to her. That was curious to me.

Phoebe's presence and attentiveness clearly offered Abby an alternative experience of relationship. Horowitz refers to dogs as 'students of behavior' (Horowitz, 2009, p. 163). They never stop looking at and studying us humans. Horowitz contends that dogs can identify characteristics of an individual through smell and nonverbal behavior and can recognize the physiological changes that accompany fear, anxiety and sadness. 'As the perpetual student, the dog knows our most ordinary of behaviors and these behaviors are chock full of information the dog can then mine' (Horowitz, 2009, pp. 166–167).

It would seem that Phoebe knew that Abby was disconnected and certainly sad. As a young dog that paid close attention to my comings and goings she, for some wonderful reason, took a particular interest in Abby. From day one, Phoebe would assume her position next to Abby on the couch, and remarkably, Abby didn't push her away. It was out of a spontaneous, and a rather desperate moment that I began to talk to Abby through Phoebe, which allowed me to 'mine' her truth, her voice. She would hardly speak unless it was to tell me something about a computer game, which felt like a time filler, an avoidance, a well-rehearsed strategy. Phoebe allowed me to puncture Abby's same-old-same-old responses.

Stern discusses Winnicott's concept of the 'transitional object' as having both intrapsychic and interpersonal qualities. The idea that an object can both contain intrapsychically and possess external and tangible qualities allow the transitional object to safely 'hold' the child and provide an environment for growth to occur. Holmes, when discussing attachment, refers to the ability of an internalized object to profoundly alter the life cycle. '[W]e need someone to be there for us—and if not a person then an animal' (1996, p. 66). Phoebe's constant presence allowed Abby to have a different experience of attachment and provided the warm and safe holding environment unique to a transitional object.

Abby certainly became more animated, and so did I, when 'Phoebe' would talk to her about something. When she drew pictures, told stories or played any computer game, Phoebe would have questions for her, a comment about what she was doing or not doing. Her disagreements with Phoebe suggested to me that there was a shift in her ability to be present, and perhaps, attach in the treatment room.

The content of Abby's statements and responses revealed a positive transference towards Phoebe. Additionally, the resulting use of Phoebe and through the nature of the play itself, Abby was able to move developmentally in her play towards being and feeling seen in the treatment room. Through imaginative play, suggest Brown and Vaughn, 'a child stops thinking about thinking. The child can then become a different self' (2009, p. 17). Additionally, they state that during play, the brain is making sense of itself. New connections and insights can form along with a shift in cognition helping to sculpt the young brain. 'For humans, creating simulations of life may be play's most valuable benefit' (ibid, p. 34). Slade and Wolf (1999) further state that 'during the first two years of life, the child undergoes a series of developmental transitions ... [T]he major cognitive achievement is the gradual emergence of the ability to represent experience symbolically, according to Piaget—into both play and language' (p. 149).

Abby was thus able to safely attach and feel a sense of belonging to such an extent that she could find her 'self' and her voice with just enough distance, through Phoebe. Brown and Vaughan state that when 'food and sleep are in peril, play will disappear' (2009, p. 42). Though, in Abby's case, lack of sleep and disinterest in eating may also have been a reflection of her disconnection and the absorption of her mother's depression. Certainly, not eating is an effective way to not be alive, and to not feel oneself. By now Abby had begun to sleep, and she then began to feel more connected during the day at school. And, little by little, she began to eat at lunch with the other children.

In order for Abby's attachment to develop into a healthier internal working model, 'she needed to be seen and known, the primary mechanism by which an infant comes to know and be known by another's mind' (Beebe and Lachmann, 2014, p. 35). Being seen in the treatment by Phoebe, then myself, and then subsequently by her mother, gave Abby an internalized structure and a developing sense that she was becoming both seen and known. Phoebe, from the beginning, saw Abby. In school, Abby began to have friends. It wasn't easy, and there were many bumps in the road, but she began to use her words without fear and spontaneously in a way that has demonstrated stunning insight.

The present

Finishing with the appointment before Abby, I heard the door to the waiting room open and a stream of giggling from her that I had never heard. It was startling because I had realized at that moment that I had never heard Abby laugh or giggle—ever. When I went out to greet Abby, with Phoebe in tow, she was laughing and giggling contagiously. She was smiling the biggest, most inviting smile I had ever seen on her face. She wanted to hurry up and come in to play. Abby has never initiated any play—other than the occasional board game. Abby's play, on those infrequent occasions, consisted of her taking a board game down, and becoming impatient with me when trying to learn and follow the rules, or realizing that she would have to work to first learn and then potentially win. This was true for all the games she had ever attempted in the sessions prior to this.

Abby looked more grown-up during this session. She was behaving in a way I had never experienced from her. She felt more engaged, determined to pick what she wanted to play and insistent on staying with her choice. She had clearly shifted emotionally and physically during this past summer. Her facial structure seemed to be changing giving her the appearance of a strikingly beautiful budding young adolescent. I found myself looking at her as though she was a different child. Coming in she insisted she measure her height with my height so we could see who was taller in a very playful and rather taunting style. She was catching up to me, she insisted. (I am all of 5'3"). Abby's measuring her height against mine felt like a statement about the internal developmental shift toward a more oedipal dynamic. Abby's comparison to me in the context of the transference allows her to reach and to grow and have an alive mother, this time. She is beginning to insist by her words and with her actions that her mother become alive.

After some playful back and forth, Abby insisted we play Twister. Though rather easy with two people, we modified the rules: one of us would be in charge of the spinner, having to label the colored circles one through six in a consistent manner and try to create a scenario where the other person would fall. Each of us had three tries, each turn. Though I could see Abby's physical lack of strength, she held her own. In the end, she out-strategized me—fair and square. I lost. She flaunted her win with that big beautiful smile. Given Abby's history around her lack of any ability to socialize, make eye contact and simply relate, this was a milestone and a moment that gave me great pause.

Discussion

Abby's treatment is now into its fifth year. She is twelve years old, entering seventh grade as a wonderfully awkward pre-adolescent who is worried about her clothes, her schoolwork and her friends. She excels in every subject and wants to be a writer when she grows up.

When Abby came in those first months, I didn't know how I could possibly gain a point of entry into this withdrawn young girl. As Phoebe relentlessly sat next to her and I sat next to Phoebe, Phoebe was then situated in the middle of the two of us. We would both pet Phoebe, but most of the time I was talking to myself until that desperate moment when I spoke to Abby through Phoebe. It was rather one-sided at first until it began to take shape as a playful kind of back and forth—the beginnings of a conversation. Every game in the room had felt off-limits to Abby. She was not interested in most things, other than the iPad or Gameboy games she brought in herself. I did not experience these games as shared play. She was expertly keeping me out of her world. Phoebe told her many things I could not have said to her. She answered Phoebe. She would get off the couch and look at Phoebe to make sure she got the message. I had no sense of hope that this was achieving anything meaningful until she began to bring in her stuffed animals from home—by the armful. When her mother was able to utilize this strategy we devised at home I felt that Abby could practice communicating in this manner, within the context of the relationship that mattered the most to her, her mother, as a true form of reparation. Her mom came in for her own sessions rather frequently as she was increasingly brought on board and taught about using the strategy of talking as if she were one of the stuffed animals, as an attempt to repair some of the damage that she felt so terribly guilty about having induced in her children. She began to get some real feedback from Abby in this process. While it was hard for her to hear the negative pushback from Abby, she worked to respond differently. When Abby became argumentative and angry, Abby's mom really struggled with how to navigate her anger without taking it personally or lashing back at her. We worked tirelessly so she could see the big picture—which she ended up understanding in theory at first. Supporting her mom to employ at home a successful way for Abby to feel heard and seen in an authentic way was a real struggle for us all.

One day, Abby cut off most of her hair. When she entered the treatment room, next time, I noticed it immediately. From my perspective, this was a statement that Abby was ready to be seen—truly. Unbeknownst to me, a fight had occurred at home because Abby did not discuss cutting her hair with her mom and stepdad before she did so. They were enraged thinking that she should have asked them first. When we discussed this together, Abby remarked to her parents, 'do you know why I didn't ask you? Because you would have said "NO!"'. Remarkably, after some discussion, her mother agreed with her. This new haircut represented another shift in Abby wanting and needing to be seen and to individuate. Seen by her classmates, her parents, the world. Seen by all.

She went to school wearing her new clothes with her new haircut. This is when she tried out for the school play. Though very tentative and self-doubting, she learned her lines and worked hard to be heard by the audience. Everyone was very proud of her. Though I could not attend the play, her mother sent me videos. Abby allowed me to watch them with her, and she narrated scene by scene what she was thinking during the performance. Her language was beginning to accurately reflect her internal world. Since Abby was an avid reader, her knowledge of the language was sitting inside of her waiting for an opportunity to be put to use—to express the luscious yet painfully lonely world that lived inside of her. As her words moved more fluently in her relationships with the other children at school, she became much more spontaneous in her actions, her play and in her interactions with human beings—adults and children alike. She was beginning to feel the warmth of connection and was devouring it like the most nourishing meal she has ever had. No wonder her entire physical structure is changing. And, that beautiful smile.

From the very beginning, on that very first day, Phoebe wanted you to know, Abby, that she has *always* believed in you.

References

Altman, N., Briggs, R., Frankel, J., Gensler, D., and Pantone, P. (2010) *Relational child psychotherapy*. New York: Other Press.

Beebe, B., and Lachmann, F.M. (2014) *The origins of attachment: Infant research and adult treatment*. New York: Routledge.

Brown, S.L. and Vaughan, C.C. (2009) *Play: How it shapes the brain, opens the imagination and invigorates the Soul*. New York: Avery.

Holmes, J. (1996) *Attachment, intimacy, autonomy: Using attachment theory in adult psychotherapy*. New York: Jason Aronson.

Horowitz, A. (2009) *Inside of a dog: What dogs see, smell and know*. New York: Scribner.

Kohon, G. (1999) *The dead mother: The work of André Green*. New York: Routledge.

Slade, A. and Wolf, D. (1999) *Children at play: Clinical and developmental approaches to meaning and representation*. New York: Oxford University Press.

Stern, D.N. (1995) *The motherhood constellation: A unified view of parent-infant psychotherapy*. New York: Basic Books/Harper Collins Publishers.

16 Countertransferential? Counter-therapeutic? Counter-intuitive? Some concluding thoughts

Jo Silbert and Jo Frasca

The abundance of material on animal-assisted therapy together with our anecdotal experiences and the increasing scientific evidence (see, in this volume, Chapters 3, 4 and 5 by Rachmani, Meggeson and Roitman, respectively) attesting to the remedial, relational and empathic qualities of animals offer us a valuable opportunity to develop a framework for thinking about how animals may be considered legitimate partners in the practice of contemporary relational psychoanalysis and psychotherapy.

As some of the contributors to this volume have suggested, discussion about the impact of animals on the practice of contemporary relational psychoanalytic psychotherapy is scant. The authors of the foregoing chapters have thus begun to address this omission in the literature by collectively considering how an animal in the clinical space may offer opportunities for the examination of the human psyche within a triadic – or group – relational matrix of which an animal is a part. By exploring, in the context of an animal's presence, principles fundamental to relational psychoanalysis, such as the analytic relationship, frame, enactments and the third, the authors demonstrate how animals may be seen as subjective others, trigger unconscious conflicts and act as a bridge connecting the various dominions of intra- and interpersonal experience.

By way of elaboration, the contributors of these chapters have shared case material and clinical thoughts emanating from their practices, often including challenges presented by working with an animal in the treatment arena. Indeed, some have shared their struggles, processes and clinical reflections behind their introduction of the animal into their treatment spaces, thereby alerting us to the myriad of factors to be thoughtfully engaged with, prior to doing so.

Along these lines, we believe that there is another matter which invites our judicious consideration. In this final chapter, we have decided to introduce into the conversation some thoughts about the sporadic inclination on the part of some animals to involuntarily mute affective expression and perhaps even banish affective experience by their propensity – surely neurobiologically designed, intuitively informed and perhaps countertransferentially driven – to comfort or soothe humans in distress. This chapter questions whether animal empathy and care thus demonstrated, in arresting affect expression, undermines the transformative potential of the psychotherapy process (Fosha, 2000, 2003) and is thus counter-therapeutic, or whether such intuitive behaviour on the part of the animal presents a unique opportunity for understanding the intrapsychic and relational worlds of the patient, and thereby facilitates the analytic work (Grossmark, 2012a, b).

The power of affect: traumatic beginnings

Trauma in early development, as a primary agent of dissociation, will impede the brain's capability to regulate in social and therapeutic settings (Schore, 2011; Bromberg, 2006, 1989). In response to traumatic circumstances, Fosha (2003) reminds us that in an attempt to restore a tenuous attachment bond, children will resort to 'defensive exclusion' (p. 228) of whatever emotions result in the volatility or reactive withdrawal of an emotionally under-resourced parent, thus undermining the development of self, self-with-other and optimal functioning in the world (Fosha, 2000).

The power of affect expression: 'charting a new course'

Difficulties acquired through experience should be transformed through experience (Fosha, 2000; Gill, in Kahn, 1991). By the psychotherapist's commitment to activities dedicated to promoting the patient's sense of safety, to actively share in the challenges of the emotional work (Grossmark, 2012b; Fosha, 2003) and to her belief in human beings' capacity to tolerate 'risk and trust …. [alongside]… suffering and despair' (Fosha, 2000, p. 6), the analytic dyad's regulatory capabilities (Grossmark, 2012b; Shane et al., 1997) and interactive process are enhanced and the patient is supported by the analytic relationship in 'charting a new course' (Fosha, ibid, p. 6).

Fosha's (2000) work on affect offers a persuasive exploration of affective experience and expression as integral to psychological transformation. She conceives of *affect* as an adaptive and complex phenomenon which reveals an individual's experiences of self, other and the intricacies of their relational patterns and *affective experience* (2003) as being integral to resourcefulness in relationships and in the world. In a conducive relational and affective milieu, patients are able to risk both expression and experience of previously disavowed traumatic, frightening and intimate emotions, paving the way for trauma recovery and the patient's emergence more fully into being and more fully in connection with an other (Fosha, 2000).

We acknowledge that not all affective expression is transformative. Fosha (2000) encourages us to distinguish between 'affective phenomena that activate deep transformational processes and other affectively-laden experiences that are not mutative' (p. 2). Rothschild (2000) alerts the psychotherapist, when the patient is in a heightened state of arousal and at risk of re-traumatisation, to the importance of titrating emotional experience and expression by 'putting on the brakes', a considered, clinically informed intervention based on attuned assessment within the context of an empathic psychotherapy relationship.

Canine countertransference

Patients may, of course, communicate defensive affects, which mask unmet longings for attachment and connection (Fosha, 2000) or unspeakable experiences, by 'impact' (Casement, 1985), potentially inducing in the psychotherapist a range of somatic, affective and/or cognitive reactions.

Saydee had learned that a person's cry is an indication of distress. At times of expression of distress during therapy, Saydee would approach some patients, one of whom we shall call K, and tap gently, repeatedly, persistently on K's foot with her paw, until K stopped crying. Be it Saydee's response to her distress at another's pain, an inability to bear her distress or a reflection of how she historically needed to protect and take care of her little owner, her gesture would have the desired effect: K seemed to excise his distress, just as he had always done.

As with Fosha's explanation above of the process of 'defensive exclusion', thus it is in the clinical space; the overt and unconscious communications between psychotherapist and patient generate an emotional environment – made no less compelling by a dog's contribution – which sanctions and vetoes certain responses and behaviours. When the therapeutic environment cannot support patients to feel safe in their affective experience and expression, they are susceptible to the defensive exclusion of the very agent – affect – which Fosha repeatedly argues is vital to their psychological growth.

K's distress clearly induced a reaction in Saydee (but it could as easily have been in the psychotherapist) that precipitated her (Saydee's, in this case) response and the patient-canine interaction that followed, apparently reinstated K's armour. Indeed, if such gestures on the part of the dog are experienced by the patient as soothing rather than intrapsychically dangerous, it must be profoundly affirming to have one's distress so deeply witnessed and attended to by a dog making deliberate physical contact. On the other hand, while, in such moments, it may be tempting for us to believe that a 'cute' intervention such as Saydee's could be comforting for a patient and that this could generate a helpful piece of cognitive work, such left brain reasoning could also bypass crucial latent material (Schore, 2011). Indeed, it could reflect a collusion with the patient's dissociative tendencies, which are designed to protect him from traumatic feelings. A sanctioning of an adaptation or a deferral to the animal's intervention may appear to be a humane act of caring, but such gestures can be a masquerade for rescuing, and as such, could hinder the psychotherapeutic process.

Fosha (2000) alerts us to the possibility that assumptions about the fragility of patients may be rationalisations for ineffective techniques and suggests that fragility should not be used to hinder clinical interventions. We are reminded here (Shane et al., 1997; Kahn, 1991) of Kohut's assertion of the therapeutic value of optimal frustration. Rather than gratification by caretaking behaviour, it may be the simultaneous experience of optimal frustration and empathy which is more likely to motivate change and growth. Notwithstanding Shane et al.'s (1997) recognition that there are some authors who believe that optimal frustration does not adequately explain development, a triadic psychotherapist/patient/dog dynamic, triggered by the dog's attempt to soothe the patient, may preclude opportunities not only for any advantages that optimal frustration might have yielded but for the intrapsychic and relational opportunities embedded in the patient's affective expression. While such caring/rescuing behaviour by an animal may be directed to the patient and appear to be an animal-patient collaboration, the psychotherapist herself – when she is unbearably impacted by the affective intensity in the room – may unconsciously recruit the dog as her proxy. She may thus also become a beneficiary of the dog's intuitive intervention – with trauma recovery, a casualty. Or would it be?

Counter-therapeutic caretaking vs clinical choice

A collision of somato-affective experience between patient and psychotherapist or between the psychotherapist's personal and professional selves may catalyse a cascade of adjunctive reactions, beginning with the removal by the psychotherapist of '"potentially objectionable" parts of [her] countertransference repertoire' (Leigh, 2011, p. 328) causing her to intervene by reactively withholding from the patient. Leigh (ibid) proposes an alternative response; that in these 'edge moments' of activation, the psychotherapist recognises that she has been impacted, applies a metaphorical 'pause button' and thus creates a space to listen deeply to the patient's coded information and process his disguised communications from within the relational matrix.

At what point, though, is the pause button to be applied? And to whom? At the moment of the dog's revelation of her intention to approach the patient? Or when the psychotherapist notices her own reaction to the dog's behaviour?

Central to contemporary relational psychoanalysis is the notion of the analytic field, an idiosyncratic analytic entity with a life of its own, both architect and artefact of the analytic encounter, which patient and analyst co-create and are organised by, and which brings the analytic couple into being. The field is distinguished by its own unconscious (Grossmark, 2012a) which does not reside inside the mind of either individual, but both crafts and emerges through dyadic interaction. The treatment itself is best served by the psychotherapist's understanding of the process as being informed by communication from the unconscious of the dyad as to the state of the relationship and by the recognition of his or her role in the emerging field (ibid).

In the unfolding of the analytic dyad's distinctive story, interactions that fully involve both psychotherapist and patient will also emerge. Such analytic occurrences offer crucial information about the analytic relationship, its participants, about what is 'un-knowable' and about the trauma that resides in the field. Such information 'can only come through "unmentalized" and "undreamable" (Ogden, 2009, p. 16) occurrences that involve patient, analyst, and the dyad's unity, the field' (Grossmark, 2012a, p. 291). Such happenings, which Grossmark refers to as 'the flow of enactive engagement' constitute therapeutic action which is to be welcomed, unobstructed, surrendered to (Grossmark, 2012b) and 'lived with and through' by the analyst (Grossmark, 2012a), thereby allowing the field to narrate its own story. Such engagements 'foster the coming to life of the patient' (Grossmark, 2012b, p. 638) and are 'the key to the therapeutic action of a contemporary psychoanalysis' (Grossmark, 2012a, p. 287).

With a dog in the room, the dyad becomes a triad and the field is accordingly authored. Patient, psychotherapist and dog now co-create and are organised by the field, the analytic relationship is expanded and "unmentalized" and "undreamable" enactment happenings now involve patient, psychotherapist, the dog and the triad. At that moment when K, placated by the Saydee's concerned tapping, withholds his affective expression, it seems evident that Saydee most certainly intervened in the patient's affective expression and experience, that she most certainly had something to do with the K's affect inhibition and that K's response was possibly a repetitive pattern. The denial to K of the opportunity to weep openly in the supportive, affirming presence of an other, may have precluded a therapeutic breakthrough. Is this, in fact, a moment of repetition? Or repair? Was a therapeutic opportunity forfeited? Or gained?

If affective experience and expression within the psychotherapy relationship are mutative and 'affective competence is the capacity to feel and deal while relating' (Fosha, 2000, p. 6), the inhibition of affect may well have been counter-therapeutic. By deciding to train *the dog* to apply the pause button so as not to intervene at such moments of affect dysregulation, we would privilege the transformative power of affect.

If, however, the dog's unimpeded intervention elicited the emergence of the patient's primitive and regressed state by which his inner world, *with* its disavowal of affect, complex needs and disorganized states could be accessed (Grossmark, 2012b), and the psychotherapist, noticing her own reactivity to the dog, applies the metaphoric pause button to *herself*, thereby unobtrusively allowing the field to narrate its own story, another key to healing may emerge (ibid). In this case, we privilege the transformative potential of the triadic interaction.

What then would be our recommendations? Perhaps to remain alert to enactments amongst and between all sentient participants who constitute the analytic triad, as well as to developmental trauma, 'the flow of enactive engagement', and to the difference between reactive caretaking, rescuing and regulating. Defensive caretaking behaviour on the part of the animal, we have seen, may arrest the process of psychotherapy. And then again, it may not.

We conclude with our recognition of those who have grappled with and been rewarded by working from a relational perspective in the presence of an animal. We offer our appreciation to those who have been open to thinking about and sharing their experiences, struggles, thoughts, stories, cautions and reflections. We acknowledge their foresight in working creatively with the analytic frame and the framework of analytic language and we wish to express our indebtedness to the animals themselves for their fertile contributions.

References

Bromberg, P. M. (1989) *Standing in the spaces: Essays on clinical process, trauma and dissociation*. Hillsdale, NJ: The Analytic Press.

Bromberg, P. M. (2006) *Awakening the dreamer: Clinical journeys*. Mahwah, NJ: The Analytic Press.

Casement, P. (1985) *On learning from the patient*. Routledge: London.

Fosha, D. (2000) *The transforming power of affect: A model for accelerated change*. New York: Basic Books.

Fosha, D. (2003) Dynamic regulation and experiential work with emotion and relatedness in trauma and disorganised attachment. In M. F. Solomon and D. J. Siegel (Eds.), *Healing trauma: Attachment, mind, body, and brain* (pp. 221–281). New York: W.W. Norton & Company, Inc.

Grossmark, R. (2012a) The flow of enactive engagement. *Contemporary Psychoanalysis*. 48(3), pp. 287–300.

Grossmark, R. (2012b). The unobtrusive relational analyst. *Psychoanalytic Dialogues*. 22(6), pp. 629–646.

Kahn, M. (1991) *Between therapist and client: The new relationship*. New York: W.H. Freeman and Company.

Leigh, E. (2011) The censorship process: From distillation to essence—A relational methodology. In H. Fowlie and C. Sills (Eds.), *Relational transactional analysis: Principles in practice* (pp. 327–336). London: Karnac.

Rothschild, B. (2000) *The body remembers: The psychophysiology of trauma and trauma treatment*. New York: W.W. Norton and Company Inc.

Shane, M., Shane, E. and Gales, M. (1997) *Intimate attachments: Toward a new self psychology*. New York: The Guilford Press.

Schore, A. N. (2011) The right brain implicit self lies at the core of psychanalysis. *Psychoanalytic Dialogues*. 21(1), pp. 75–100.

Index

For Product Safety Concerns and Information please contact our EU
representative GPSR@taylorandfrancis.com
Taylor & Francis Verlag GmbH, Kaufingerstraße 24, 80331 München, Germany

www.ingramcontent.com/pod-product-compliance
Lightning Source LLC
Chambersburg PA
CBHW070334270326
41926CB00017B/3862

9 780367 437800